Doctors Serving People

Critical Issues in Health and Medicine

Edited by Rima D. Apple, University of Wisconsin–Madison, and Janet Golden, Rutgers University, Camden

Growing criticism of the U.S. health care system is coming from consumers, politicians, the media, activists, and health care professionals. Critical Issues in Health and Medicine is a collection of books that explores these contemporary dilemmas from a variety of perspectives, among them political, legal, historical, sociological, and comparative, and with attention to crucial dimensions such as race, gender, ethnicity, sexuality, and culture.

Doctors Serving People

Restoring Humanism to Medicine through Student Community Service

Edward J. Eckenfels

Rutgers University Press

New Brunswick, New Jersey, and London

Library of Congress Cataloging-in-Publication Data

Eckenfels, Edward J.
Doctors serving people : restoring humanism to medicine through student community
service / Edward J. Eckenfels.
   p. ; cm.—(Critical issues in health and medicine)
  Includes bibliographical references and index.
  ISBN 978–0-8135–4315–4 (hardcover : alk. paper)
  ISBN 978–0-8135–4316–1 (pbk. : alk. paper)
  1. Community health services—United States. 2. Student volunteer in medical care—
United States. I. Title, II. Series.
  [DNLM: 1. Community Health Services—United States. 2. Community Networks—
United States: 3. Social Responsibility—United States. 4. Students, Medical—
United States. WA 546 AA1 E19d 2008
  RA445.E26 2008
  362.12—dc22   2007037881

A British Cataloging-in-Publication record for this book is available from the British Library.

Visit our Web site: http://rutgerspress.rutgers.edu

Manufactured in the United States of America

Contents

Foreword

Early on in my position as Dean of Student Affairs at Dartmouth Medical School, I was asked to bring a group of our medical students to meet with Dr. Robert Coles over breakfast. Dr. Coles, the noted author and child psychiatrist, professor of medicine and humanities at Harvard, and recipient of the Pulitzer Prize for his work in documenting the experiences of those children first involved in the integration of the schools in the South, was giving Dartmouth's fall convocation speech that day. Dr. Coles and I lingered after the breakfast meeting with the students and talked about our dreams for and worry about medical education. We developed a friendship, a lasting bond, and he became my mentor. I, in turn, became convinced that his approach of participating in direct service to a community combined with using literature as a means of provoking reflection was a very useful strategy for education, especially the education of medical students. Dr. Coles's important books *The Call of Stories: Literature and the Moral Imagination* (1990) and *The Call of Service: A Witness to Idealism* (1994), became my guidebooks and his approach of "doing as a part of learning" became my mantra.

Over the years, I witnessed how Dr. Coles's stories could light a fire with students (and probably even more so with me). One story I'll never forget was about his mentor, Erik Erikson. Once in a class at Harvard, Dr. Erikson asked his students if they had any questions for him. There was a silence, but finally, a young woman with a soft voice in the middle of the room asked him, "What do you think a Harvard education should mean when it's all over?" Dr. Erikson smiled and said, "That's a big question—an important one." After a thoughtful pause, he answered, "I hope this is a place where we can all grow ethically— where we become kinder and more thoughtful toward others." He paused again and said, "All the knowledge in the world is but a prelude to the moral challenges of our everyday life." Dr. Coles reflected that "we all need to struggle on behalf of a life in which daily deeds measure up to professed pieties." This same type of question could be asked of medical education: what is its purpose? The glib answer might be to produce the types of doctors that society wants and needs, ones who can attend to our health and advocate for better health care. But is this what we're producing? I think in large part the answer is no. How could this be so? If so, how can it be changed?

A common question being asked at present is what has become of the concept of professionalism in medicine, airing a concern that we have lost our bearings. Much attention in the medical education literature and a significant amount of time at medical meetings is currently being devoted to trying to define this concept of professionalism and figuring out ways to teach and evaluate it. In the most widely accepted definition, experts agree that society cedes medical professionals many privileges, but also in return, expects certain obligations, the most important of which is to respond to the society's health needs. Many are worried that we are not meeting these obligations and calls from leadership urge medicine to "return to its core values" as a profession, or to "reestablish" its covenant with society. But why should we have to "return to" or "reestablish" these things? What is happening and why? Has something been lost? What is in jeopardy with this state of affairs?

One of the most compelling articles I have ever read about the reasons for this situation was called "Structure and Ideology in Medical Education: An Analysis of Resistance to Change," by the great medical sociologist Samuel Bloom. Bloom seemed to hit the nail on the head when he stated that "the scientific mission of academic medicine has crowded out its social responsibility to train for society's most basic health care delivery needs . . . medical education's manifest humanistic mission is little more than a screen for the research mission which is the major concern of the institution's social structure." Indeed, Bloom (1988) suggested that "education is a minor mission of medical schools" where research is king and the structure of the system is to foster innovation and discovery. In 2005, the noted medical historian Dr. Kenneth Ludmerer (2004) identified another important theme, that is, that the business and clinical revenue issue, "the bottom line" mentality, was the second important driver of the system, making education and responding to societal needs even more marginalized.

Just about any account or media depiction of the immersion of medical students into this milieu, beginning with the study by Howard Becker in 1961 of the experiences of students at the University of Kansas detailed in the book *Boys in White* (Becker et al. 2002), all indicate that idealism is an early casualty for students as they band together against the system. Students often experience a confusing atmosphere of mixed messages in their training and a test-strewn, competitive, judgmental, and lonely educational environment that inhibits idealism, is full of instances of shame and humiliation, and has been facetiously called the precynical and cynical years. Many find these last descriptors closer to the truth than they want to believe. One of my colleagues at Dartmouth always admonishes, "Every system is perfectly designed to get the results it gets"; and I once heard a colleague say that "the most common outcome of the heavy science curriculum is to get the students to hate science."

Dr. Coles describes this phenomenon eloquently in his essay "The Moral Education of Medical Students" (2003). He says:

> To be sure factual information counts a lot; we have to impart it constantly, and our students are mightily challenged as they absorb blackboards full of information, textbooks full of explanations, and as they try to keep in mind what they have learned in long laboratory sessions. All too often, though, those students will wonder what the point of such an experience is . . . and they will resort to gastrointestinal imagery as they try to gain any possible perspective on a relentlessly demanding, exhausting, unnerving experience: ingestion, regurgitation. . . . Some medical schools have tried hard to emphasize ideas and ways of thinking so that an ever-expanding mass of detailed information can be fitted to broad understanding of how things work in our bodies. Of course such efforts of reform have to contend with the so-called Boards, the gateway to certification for state licensing. And so, despite curricular reforms, medical students still have to cram and cram in order to get through multiple-choice tests that are not exactly designed to do justice to the complexity of things, nor to encourage independent or reflective thinking. Indeed, in medicine especially, with its emphasis on human particularity and on individual idiosyncrasy (the old adage "each patient is different"), the use of multiple-choice tests, with their frequent emphasis on yes and no, right or wrong, is both ironic and not likely to encourage medical students to think broadly, make connections across various academic fields of inquiry, or develop any kind of wide-ranging, open-eyed responsiveness to patients in all their puzzling, surprising variation. . . . I mention such familiar aspects of medical school education because they are not without moral implications. Students are told to stuff their heads with information, the more obscure, the more likely to be queried, students are told they are in a rock-bottom sense competing against one another on one "curve" after another, are not encouraged to think about the truly consequential or do so in alliance with one another. (55–58)

What are we to do?

Reflecting on these types of issues is how I first met Edward Eckenfels. I run the New Hampshire–Vermont Albert Schweitzer Fellowship and Ed has been involved since the outset in the Chicago-based program. The fellowship selects young professionals for projects to attack unmet health needs. Each Schweitzer fellow does two hundred hours of direct service connected to a supporting agency, so it will be sustained; meets with the other fellows monthly to help each other along; and works with the group to produce community symposia. The program is founded on the ideals of Dr. Schweitzer, who said to young people, "Grow into your ideals so that life can never rob you of them." Ed and I were at a program directors' retreat in a beautiful inn in Kennebunkport, Maine, and it was here I first heard and marveled at the Rush Community Service Initiatives Program. Ed is a street-smart, and a passionate, visionary and an inspiring grassroots activist and leader. His approach to medical education was nurtured by things like Freedom Summer, the push for voter registration in Mississippi. He has learned by experience how to work with underserved communities. He convinced me that the Rush program was special, and with every accumulating detail he told me about, I became more and more convinced he had to write this book. I suspect it is my cheerleader mentality that caused him to approach me about writing this foreword. I have seen the letters of support for Ed's work by such luminaries as C. Everett Koop, Jordan Cohen, Tom Inui, Bud Baldwin, Fred Hafferty, Tracy Kidder, Robert Coles, and others who would surely have jumped at the opportunity to write this and so I feel humbled and hope my words will do justice to how important I feel this work is.

Doctors Serving People: Restoring Humanism to Medicine through Student Community Service is a story of courage, vision, and empowerment. It is a story of one of our greatest cities, the "city with the big shoulders," "the hog butcher of the world"—Chicago—and Ed beautifully lays out the issues that come with urbanization, things Paul Farmer would call examples of "structural violence" (such as the Henry Horner housing project) that set the physical and sociocultural milieu that becomes such a barrier to good health. Indeed, within the dysfunctional U.S. health care system, of which Chicago is a microcosm, studies of health outcomes have shown that there are actually "eight Americas," with the health care at the top stratum equal to the best in the world, but the care at the lowest equal to the worst care anywhere. Longevity in the United States varies widely, from Asian American women in Bergen County, New Jersey, who live to an average age of ninety-one—three years longer than women in Japan (the country with the highest female life expectancy)—to Native American men in South Dakota, who live only fifty-eight years on average, a lifespan akin to that of men in Azerbaijan. Young and middle-aged blacks in high-risk urban areas have mortality risks closer to those in the Russian Federation or parts of sub-Saharan Africa than to those in neighboring white suburbs. Despite efforts to reduce racial and ethnic health inequalities in recent years, the longevity gaps within the U.S. population have remained virtually unchanged for more than two decades (Institute of Medicine 2002). One's first instinct is to attribute the causes of excess mortality at younger ages to violence and HIV, but the fact is that the same old chronic diseases that affect the rest of the populations run rampant in these areas too. Just as Ed and his students have done, we need to focus on alleviating the disparities that lead to poor preventative measures and poor treatment of the most common diseases.

It is fitting that these efforts are promoted in a school named for Dr. Benjamin Rush, a physician, patriot, and signer of the Declaration of Independence. The students at the school named for him are trying to enact the vision of the founding fathers of life, liberty, and happiness for all. The school is living the vision of Woodrow Wilson, who as president of Princeton said, "It's not learning but service that will give a college a place in the public annals of the nation." Or Ira Harkavy of the Center for Community Partnerships of the University of Pennsylvania, who said, "Universities can no longer afford to remain shores of affluence, self-importance and horticultural beauty at the edge of inland seas of squalor, violence, and despair." Ed and the Rush students are doing something special to "return" to our values and "reestablish" our covenant with society. A recent popular book called *The Devil in the White City* details the story of Chicago during the time of the 1893 World's Fair (Larson 2004). The "devil" is a hideous, psychopathic murderer, who happens also to be a doctor. I would suggest that Ed be considered the "angel" in the White City, someone who brings hope, support, guidance, and inspiration.

One of the books that Dr. Coles uses as a mainstay in his Harvard courses is James Agee and Walker Evans's *Let Us Now Praise Famous Men* (1960). This is a photodocumentary of the plight of sharecroppers in the South. Agee, in a no-holds-barred, in-your-face way, challenges the readers: "Now that you've seen this, what are you going to do?" That's the way I'd suggest the readers approach this current inspiring story about this innovative program. What are *you* going to do with this provocative piece of work, this successful experiment called the Rush Community Service Initiatives Program? Tracy Kidder's book about Paul Farmer, *Mountains beyond Mountains* (2003), has inspired many to fight against structural violence and for health equity. This book should inspire a similar reaction. By implanting it or parts of it into medical education, perhaps there can be innovation *with* change, a return to our core values and the covenant we are supposed to have with society. Perhaps participants "learning by doing" about health system barriers, anthropology, epidemiology, the socio-cultural determinants of health, and many more subjects could become activists to change our dysfunctional health care system, to strive for health equity, to eliminate those eight levels of health care in America, and to better address the inequities in health in the world.

But above all I feel that this is a book for leaders. Those chroniclers of history Will and Ariel Durant wrote a short book called *The Lessons of History* (1993). In it, they said, "When a group or a civilization declines, it is through no mystic limitation of corporate life but through the failure of its political and intellectual leaders to meet the challenge of change."

This book shows a path to meet those challenges.

Joseph F. O'Donnell, MD
Senior Advising Dean and Director of
Community Programs
Dartmouth Medical School
Hanover, New Hampshire

Acknowledgments

There are so many people who have helped and supported me, it is impossible to acknowledge all of them. There are, however, a few individuals without whose personal commitment it would have been extremely difficult to make the Rush Community Service Initiatives Program (RCSIP) a reality.

Top medical center administrators who backed us from the beginning included Leo Henikoff, MD, during his tenure as president and CEO; Erich Brueschke, MD, during the time he was dean of the medical school; and Larry Goodman, MD, as associate dean of Medical Students Programs, as dean, and, currently, as CEO and president. James A. Schoenberger, MD, chairman of the Department of Preventive Medicine, and his successor, Henry Black, MD, gave us office space, access to copying, and personal support and encouragement. The entire Office of Philanthropy and Communication got us off to a good start by finding potential sources of funding, but we owe special thanks to Carol Covington and Patty Shea. Max Brown, general counsel for the medical center, provided legal advice (including hiring a law student to work with us) so we could address the malpractice issue. Margaret McLaughlin, MD, assistant dean for Career Counseling, gave us the data for our analysis of academic performance.

Dr. Steven Daughtery, a whiz of a biostatistician and social psychologist, did all the statistical analysis in our study of the relationship between the extent of student participation and their academic performance and residency selection. Amy Valukus, who served as the third program director, was not only outstanding in her coordination but also instrumental in initiating the school-based clinic project.

Through his empathy, receptiveness, and willingness to go the extra mile, Dr. Paul Jones, who took over the directorship of RCSIP when I retired, kept the RCSIP spirit alive and flourishing. Perhaps most important, he turned the daily operation of the program over to Sharon Gates, who is so much loved by the students that it makes me jealous.

DeWitt "Bud" Baldwin, MD, and Tom Inui, MD, who were kind enough to read earlier drafts, gave me invaluable recommendations on how to improve the manuscript. Fred Hafferty, PhD, who is quoted throughout the book, was my intellectual anchor. I built upon many of his ideas pertaining to the culture of medical education, and his hidden-curriculum concept was the springboard for my idea of a peripheral curriculum. Along with Bud, Tom, and Fred, Jordan Cohen, MD, C. Anderson "Andy" Hedberg, MD, and Arthur Kaufman, MD, wrote wonderful letters of support. I am deeply honored that Joseph "Joe" O'Donnell, MD, accepted my invitation to write the foreword. He stood by me through the peaks and valleys of trying to put in words what I thought, saw, and felt.

From the bottom of my heart I want to thank all the clinic directors; the Boys and Girls Club at Henry Horner; the neighborhood community centers, shelters, and health fair sponsors; and especially the students and faculty of Rush Medical College. Without their assistance and vision, RCSIP would still be an idea whose time had not come.

Finally, while Claudia and I have shared the pleasure of our work equally, I was the one obsessed with writing this book. Without her support and devotion, however, this book would never have been possible. I dedicate the book to her.

Doctors Serving People

Introduction

Humanism in the Time of Technocracy

> By any indicator—the appearance of new essays, research, curricula, feedback instruments, or innovation in certification and continued learning—in this past decade there has been a remarkable intensification of interest in professionalism in medicine.
>
> —Thomas Inui, "Educating for Professionalism in Medicine"

Can Medicine Redeem Itself?

To paraphrase the great American Revolutionary hero Thomas Paine, these are times that try the soul of American medicine.[1] Cost estimates of $2.2 trillion and rising, at least 45 million people uninsured at any given time, and mounting dissatisfaction with the quality of care received have made the existing crisis in medicine increasingly alarming. Added to the rapidly expanding list of medicine's woes are a growing physician shortage (or maldistribution and over-specialization); a leveling-off of minority admissions to medical school; a steady decline in medical school graduates seeking a career in primary care; proposed higher premiums for Medicare beneficiaries; a market-incentive health care system; for-profit HMOs; powerful health insurance lobbies; and the escalating influence of the pharmaceutical industry in the training, management, and practice of medicine.

Leaders in medicine and their respective organizations have looked inward for solutions. Since the mid-1990s, reports from the major medical organizations, essays by authorities in the health care field, and articles in the foremost professional journals have concentrated on ways to address these problems. The main focus of attention has been *professionalism*. This concern has brought forth a flood of commentary addressing a search for a conceptual yet substantive meaning of medicine as a profession.[2]

In the piece quoted above, in which he offers his viewpoint, Thomas Inui (2004), an innovative medical educator, underscores "the ideal attributes and behaviors of a virtuous person in medicine, attributes [such as respect, compassion, honesty, and ethical probity] that reflect the foundational values of the profession." A concern for identifying core values in medicine is not new. For example, Steven Schroeder (1992), a recognized expert on medical professionalism and former president of the Robert Wood Johnson Foundation, lists service, compassion, and dedication as medicine's core values and proposes that "helping those who are ill, are suffering or at risk for ill health [is] noble and enduring" (590). Renee Fox and Judith Swazey (1984), two leading scholars of medicine as a social institution, hold that such values as "decency, kindness, sympathy, empathy, caring, devotion, service, generosity, altruism, sacrifice, and love" are downplayed, and they call for a more "virtue-based" medicine (339).

Eliot Freidson (1970), the recognized sociologist on the subject, initially identified three tenets that make medicine a profession: autonomy from external assessment, control over how future physicians are trained, and sole responsibility for certification. As he dug deeper, he found that corresponding to these traits was an emerging sense of dominance and self-aggrandizement that begins early in medical school. Writing on Freidson's conceptualization more than twenty-five years later, Delese Wear (1997) observed that this professional autonomy can lead to "insularity and a self-deceiving vision of the objectivity and reliability of its knowledge and the virtues of its members" (1058).

With respect to the professional relationship between the doctor and the patient, Jodi Halpern (1993), a psychiatrist with a strong interest in empathy, believes that "the notion that *experiencing* emotion is necessary to accurately understand someone challenges the ideal of 'detached concern'" (163). She further points out that clinical empathy is frowned on because physicians are erroneously taught that it detracts from their clinical objectivity.

This renewed emphasis on reform from within medicine has a long history. The acknowledged landmark for serious medical education reform is the 1910 Flexner Report.[3] Using the Johns Hopkins University School of Medicine as his prototype, Flexner revolutionized a disorganized, chaotic apprenticeship system into a highly academic set of standards for admission, education, and graduation that the vast majority of existing schools could not meet. Although he is credited with creating a single standard of medical education based on scientific knowledge and clinical practice, Flexner is less often acknowledged for recommending that medical education meet *societal needs* and get away from being a proprietary enterprise. In this respect, he referred to the physician as a "social instrument . . . whose function is fast becoming social and preventive, rather than individual and curative."

In the 1990s Nicholas Christakis, a physician and sociologist, performed a content analysis on nineteen of twenty-four reports that directly addressed undergraduate medical education, beginning with the Flexner Report. He found four consistent objectives of reform; most often cited was serving the public interest, followed by making sure there were enough physicians, keeping up with the knowledge and skill explosion, and expanding the emphasis on generalist training. He also discovered consistency in the methods for meeting these objectives—the manner and content of the teaching, the development of a competent faculty capable of doing the job, and a willingness to pursue new ways to improve the organizational system of training. He identified three possible explanations for the similarity: the problems are viewed as inherently irremediable, but he did away with this point quickly; efforts at reform have been inadequate, although he pointed out that society changes rapidly; and medical education has made some significant changes in response. The most important explanation for him was "the affirmation of certain core professional values and the self-regulation of the profession." But Christakis (1995b) is cautious about the latter and "encourages a healthy skepticism about the potential for change in response to reform proposals" (711).

In the conclusion to his 1995 monograph, Christakis (1995a) states:

> This relative neglect of the students flows mostly from the emphasis that the reports place on patient care and research—rather than education— as the chief missions of medical schools. Indeed, the reports are relatively faceless. Despite occasional concerns with the life of students and faculty at medical schools, the reports tend to ignore the centrality of these groups in medical education. Only rarely do the reports refer directly to student or faculty concerns or to the duty owed by medical schools not so much to society-at-large but to their students. The reports are primarily concerned with other—albeit important—needs of the profession and society. (47)

For a more radical approach I turn to Sam Bloom, who almost twenty years ago wrote in his classic article "Structure and Ideology in Medical Education: An Analysis of Resistance to Change" (1988) that "the scientific mission of the academic health center has crowded out its social responsibility to train for society's health needs" (294). In an astute examination of the profession, he recognized that the proposed reforms in medical education were smoke screens for protecting the traditional curriculum from change. Furthermore, he found, "educational values become subordinate to the requisites of the *organizational* structure of the medical school" (296; italics added). Delese Wear (1997), who has analyzed contemporary medical education with a humanist's eye, also reminds us that the constant pressure to generate external funding for their research, to sustain their own salaries through clinical practice, and to keep up with the barrage of bureaucratic regulations and paperwork is stressful and demoralizing.

In 1994 Fredric Hafferty and Ronald Franks published their article, "The Hidden Curriculum, Ethics Teaching, and the Structure of Medical Education," in *Academic Medicine,* which has become a modern classic. They argue persuasively that medical schools actually have three curricula: the *formal,* which contains the stated, intended, and officially offered and endorsed teaching goals and objectives; the *informal,* which is the learning that takes place at the level of personal interaction usually initiated by a potential faculty-mentor; and the *hidden,* which is how students learn to adapt to the pressures, stresses, and social expectations of becoming a doctor. It is in this last sphere that the values, beliefs, and behaviors are cultivated and internalized.

John Evans (1992), one of the original architects of Health of the Public, a program dedicated to advancing a "population perspective" through community partnerships, curricular reform, and collaboration among health professionals, focused on the need to incorporate demand-side thinking in medical education by taking into account public expectations, the health needs of the community, and societal trends, all necessary if medicine is to sustain public trust.[4]

In response to the growing concern about losing its moral compass, the Association of American Medical Colleges convened a blue-ribbon committee of medical educators to determine the attributes that physicians should possess to practice medicine at the beginning of the twenty-first century and the contribution that the medical school experience should make to the acquisition of these attributes. The result was the report of the Medical School Objectives Project (1998; cited as MSOP), containing a series of learning objectives that were organized into four overarching precepts: a physician must be knowledgeable, must be skillful, must be altruistic, and must be dutiful. The report soon gained a lot of attention, for two reasons: first, instead of the usual subjunctive *should,* used in previous reports, the imperative *must* was emphasized; second, the inclusion of altruism and duty, which are outside the established biomedical paradigm, stressed the need to cultivate the core values of the profession.

It is my contention that over the past two decades there has been a subtle but definite disengagement from the core professional values as the foundation of medical education and a greater emphasis on the acquisition of technical knowledge and procedural skills. Hafferty (1998) has studied this change and warned, "Until we come to accept that medical training is, at root, a process of moral enculturation and that medical schools function as moral communities, the reform that is needed—the reform that the public deserves—will remain both elusive and enigmatic" (406).

This clash between the moral imperative of medicine as a humanistic call to serve and the reality of accelerating costs, limited access, and declining perceptions of quality care has led to a kind of schizoid state, with the physician caught between the daily routines required to deliver the latest advances in health care and the intrinsic values fundamental to education and practice. This is a continuing source of conflict, tension, and antagonism, but at the same time it serves to sustain the current system because clinical research, technical procedures, cost containment, and open competition in the market push a compassionate, empathetic, and holistic view of health to the sidelines. Furthermore, there is a growing tendency in medicine toward what Charles Taylor (1992), the pragmatist and humanist, calls "instrumental reason . . . that forgets the patient as a person, that takes no account of how the treatment relates to his or her story and thus the determinants of hope and despair, that neglects the essential rapport between care-giver and patient" (106).

Over a thirty-year career, I have seen this growing schism between medicine as *science* and medicine as *service*. Likewise, as Wear (2003) has shown, a once-cherished concern about how social, economic, and cultural factors affect the health of the public is rapidly diminishing. In short, American medicine has lost its connectedness to society and, in the process, has become self-absorbed, devoted more to its own technology and what it is able to do than to what patients and society actually need.

The irony of this is that by its very nature medicine is humanistic. In the course of human history, medicine's role has always been to heal illness and alleviate suffering. It attracts idealistic people, those who are dedicated to pursuing these noble beliefs. *Idealism* is the fountainhead of medicine. It is the basic attribute that draws particular individuals who are willing to devote their lives to taking care of people. For today's medical students, Paul Farmer, a medical anthropologist and infectious disease specialist who started Partners in Health and whose clinical responsibilities span three continents, is the ultimate example.[5] When Tracy Kidder, a Pulitzer Prize–winning author, asked what drives a man to such superhuman efforts, Farmer replied, "The problem is if I don't work this hard, someone will die who doesn't have to." But as for personal motivation, he goes on to say, "If you are making sacrifices, unless you're automatically following some rule, it stands to reason that you are trying to lessen some psychic discomfort. So, for example, if I took steps to be a doctor for those who don't have medical care, it could be regarded as a sacrifice, but it could be regarded as a way to deal with ambivalence. . . . I feel ambivalent about selling my services in a world where some can't buy them. You can feel ambivalent about that, because you should feel ambivalent" (Kidder 2003, 191). Clearly, not everyone can be a Paul Farmer, but the inward clarity and honesty he displays is an example to be articulated, discussed, and manifested in contemporary medical education.

Let This Little Light Shine

My primary purpose for writing this book is to provide another take on how to address these concerns. This idea didn't just occur to me. A little background should help to explain my conviction. I was a graduate student at the University of Chicago in the early 1960s. One of the wonderful things about the Chicago campus at that time was the intellectual atmosphere that was relentlessly pursuing "the nature of human nature." As someone who initially studied philosophy, particularly the post-Enlightenment thinkers who emphasized freedom, democracy, and liberalism, I was becoming more and more intrigued by the *social* sciences as an empirical way of addressing this question. I was interested in *humans,* not rats in a maze, conditioned responses, or Skinner boxes (operative conditioning chambers created by B. F. Skinner to examine animal and eventually human behavior).

During these early years at Chicago, I was deeply influenced by C. Wright Mills's magnificent book *The Sociological Imagination* (1959). What really got me was that the sociological imagination wasn't only for sociologists, but for everyone. It provided a perspective, an understanding of who you are in society. Mills characterized it as the relationship between autobiography—who I think I am—and panhistory—how events that I may not even be aware of continue to shape my identity and, I, in turn, even without my conscious awareness, shape history. It is this interconnection between self and society that I was attracted to.

From the beginning I viewed sociology as a science.[6] But I never saw it as being in the same realm as the physical sciences, with their mathematical certainty and rigorous experimental design. For me, sociology, following the reasoning of pragmatists William James and John Dewey, and articulated beautifully by Peter Berger in his marvelous little book *An Invitation to Sociology* (1963), is concerned about the ability "to discover human values that are endemic to scientific procedures in both the social and natural sciences. Such values are humility before the immense richness of the world one is investigating, an effacement of oneself in the search for understanding, honesty and precision in method, respect for findings honestly arrived at, patience and a willingness to be proven wrong, and, last but not least, the *community of other individuals* sharing these values" (166; italics added).

As a graduate student in the Department of Sociology, I became interested in the field of collective behavior—crowds, mass gatherings, political rallies, and the like. I was intrigued by social movements—people binding themselves together for a cause. I became attracted to aggregates that were dedicated to real reform, not just change for its own sake. At that time the Cold War was growing colder between the United States and the Soviet Union; the two powers had the capability to destroy each other, along with the rest of the world. An anti–nuclear war attitude was beginning to ferment among a broad spectrum of the American people. A peace movement was taking root. I was intrigued to see if it might take on the characteristics of a serious social movement, one that could result in real reform to stop the threat of nuclear war. I wrote my first paper, with Lawrence Landry (1962), about this phenomenon for the special peace issue of a radical student journal, *New University Thought*.[7]

The notion of change and reform through social action was to stick with me and spur me on throughout not simply my career but my entire life. These values were manifested and acted upon in all aspects of my later involvement in medical education and training as a teacher, researcher, counselor, administrator, and spokesperson.

On the basis of the reputation I gained teaching nursing students while I was still a graduate student, Dr. Mark Lepper, the first dean of the reactivated Rush Medical College, hired me as a special assistant in 1970.[8] Dr. Lepper was a visionary in a great many ways. Behavioral science, as a new discipline coming out of psychology, had already found its place in the medical center primarily as a testing and assessment mechanism. Dr. Lepper, trained in infectious disease and preventive medicine and with a strong bent toward social determinants of disease and illness, urged me to go to England to observe how medical sociology was being taught in the new community-based medical schools. On my return I learned that my faculty appointment was to be in the Department of Preventive Medicine, where he thought I could be most effective. This is when my career in the field of health care really began.

Dr. Lepper was instrumental in getting me involved in two major projects that provided the precedents for my position on health care and medical education. The first was a mass screening for hypertension, funded by the Office of Economic Opportunity, in Mile Square in the shadow of Chicago's West Side medical center.[9] The other was a biosocial assessment of a poor black, rural community—Holmes County, Mississippi (Eckenfels 1976).[10] By immersing myself in these two communities, one urban and one rural, I gained a new sensitivity and awareness of the importance of full partnerships with the community if essential change is to be accomplished. These studies secured my role in preventive medicine as a researcher and teacher.

In the early stages of the medical school, I also built a reputation as someone the students felt they could talk to, and so the new dean asked me if I would serve as an ombudsman on his behalf. This position allowed me to see how students attempted to deal with the stress of medical school. Later I was made an assistant dean for student counseling and in 1984 I established a faculty advisor program. My motto, taken from Gordon Allport (1962), one of the early creative minds of personality theory, was "An [advisor] is like a philosopher and friend, he loves knowledge and his fellow man" (380). In all these endeavors, I never lost sight of my interests as a researcher. Out of the advisor program evolved a longitudinal study of students' adaptation to medical school. Following this stage of my tenure at Rush, I became the director for a series of courses offered by the Department of Preventive Medicine. The challenge was to introduce the students to the importance of social factors as determinants in the health and well-being of individual patients, communities, populations, and society at large. My approach integrated epidemiological, demographic, behavioral, and cultural factors into an ecological model. There were also other topics introduced into this sequence, such as health and poverty, epidemiology and biostatistics, and community health. It was on this basis that I sent students out of the medical center and into inner-city health centers and neighborhood clinics to see, face to face, how health care was provided to the poor and disadvantaged.

These experiences were the origin of the Rush Community Service Initiatives Program (RCSIP). The construct was *service-learning,* which has become a popular term in the lexicon of medical student community service programs. Like other such dualities, it has many interpretations. The one that best fits my perspective is that of the eminent child psychiatrist, and author of the Children of Crisis series, Robert Coles (1993): the "call of service . . . results in learning about the life lived by giving freely of oneself." This book is dedicated to that proposition. It is the story of one particular community service program, but it has important implications for medicine in general and other professions with clear fiduciary and social responsibilities.

What makes RCSIP different from the more conventional service-learning programs is that, first, it is *student generated* and *student governed*. This fact is fundamental to what the program means to the student participants. They started it, and the program *belongs* to them. Second, it is completely *voluntary;* that is, there is no academic credit. Finally, it is outside the formal curriculum, which affirms its *extracurricular* status. In this regard, RCSIP thrives by its own volition because it was created by the students from scratch; it attracts students (and faculty) who volunteer to help the disadvantaged; it is a source of creativity whereby fresh minds from new classes invent or reinvent programs; and it continues by its own momentum, allowing students to participate (with faculty support) throughout all four years of medical school and, in some cases, into residency training.

These four factors—student generated, student governed, voluntary, and extracurricular—serve as the bedrock of the program. Taken together, they create a social environment—a *culture*—for fostering the growth and development (in conjunction with the knowledge and skills) of the student participants. The substance and form of the learning and development are engendered *in the community* through social action. Collectively, outside the formal medical school structure, the participants can interact openly and without trepidation among themselves and with those they serve. Ethical and humane issues can be addressed without embarrassment. Commitments are espoused. They learn medicine without fear of failing and in direct relation to a human being seeking care. Leadership evolves naturally. They realize that expensive tests and high-tech procedures may not be necessary, and in the process they become sensitive to the struggles of the poor and disadvantaged. They experience, at first hand, the distribution of health and illness in a population. They see the patient in the context of his or her culture and social circumstances. They are not afraid to be empathetic or compassionate if it doesn't distract from the medical care needed. They become more politically aware and, in some cases, radicalized. In sum, their clinical knowledge and skills, strengthened by cultural and social awareness, become tools for being humanistic in the care and treatment of the sick, regardless of race, ethnicity, and social class.

These attributes cannot be overstated. RCSIP offers another important element in understanding medicine in terms of the new sense of uncertainty that surrounds the profession. Since the turn of the twenty-first century there has been a voluminous output of writing about medicine by physician-authors. Atul Gawande (2002), a surgeon and outspoken interpreter of the current medical system, and Jerome Groopman (2007), an oncologist and one of the world's leading researchers in cancer and AIDS, both of whom write for *The New Yorker,* have published two critically acclaimed books about the current state of medicine with particular emphasis on how doctors practice and on their inability to recognize their errors. Using RCSIP as a case study, I focus primarily on a central issue that these two writers allude to, namely, the health of the public.

The RCSIP experiences, and the construct developed to facilitate them, take place in the real world, not the taken-for-granted one that insulates those who function exclusively inside the academic health center. It is in the world of poverty and deprivation that the Rush students and their faculty mentors work. Such experiences humanize medicine and all the other social endeavors for them and those they serve. What makes this particularly meaningful is that it is *their* community service program, and as such it possesses a cachet that eludes the formal structure. The personal effort and emotional energy it took to make RCSIP a reality distinguishes it from more conventional programs. The collective action of faculty and students unified them on a very basic and most human level. This is why they have held on to it with such tenacity that their stance eventually led the medical center administration to recognize RCSIP as a legitimate, permanent part of the medical school, one that it accepts but does not own. I can't think of a better example of the power of students' commitment as a force for change.

Moreover, in the process of witnessing RCSIP's evolution, the struggles and obstacles it faced, its accomplishments, and its sustainability, I saw what was *missing* in contemporary medical education, not in a technical or procedural way, but as a moral endeavor and RCSIP's implications for humanistic reform. My tracking of the program reinforced my conviction that the best way to cultivate humanistic values and develop an understanding of how sociocultural factors influence health and illness is through experiential learning. Richard Horton, editor in chief of the *Lancet,* medical journalist, and activist against the war in Iraq, in the preface of his book, *Health Wars: On the Global Front Lines of Modern Medicine* (2003), explains that health issues are deemed "soft news" by highbrow commentators on our culture "partly because health and disease are interpreted as a matter of *lifestyle* and not—as they are—profoundly existential, public policy, and geopolitical concerns" (xiv; italics added).

I begin this book by describing the genesis of RCSIP and depicting the establishment of four sets of programs initiated in the 1990s: free community-based medical clinics, AIDS-awareness projects, grassroots community-based non-medical endeavors, and health care commitments in developing countries. Narratives from student activists who are now practicing physicians, with the additional perspectives of community representatives, the faculty, and the program directors add a personal dimension.

I address the issue of evaluation theoretically and practically with emphasis on what student participants have learned, intellectually and morally, providing empirical estimates of patients and clients served. The constructs I develop throughout the book and use as the basis for promoting student idealism make it possible for me to reframe medical education as a catalyst to promote the health of the public in light of the growing movement toward some form of universal health care, the reentry of prevention as a cost-effective measure, and the need for training culturally sensitive physicians to address the requirements of our growing diverse population. Finally, I look at the current state of the program and a perspective based on my personal involvement.

In short, this little book is a big undertaking, and it is hoped that by the end I have provided the reader, in a consistent and holistic way, some sense of what Rush students have done to enhance their idealism and cultivate their humanism—a valuable lesson for us all.

Chapter 1

The Emergence of the Rush Community Service Initiatives Program

The only lost cause is one we give up on before we enter the struggle.	I think we learn . . . that the call of service is a call towards others—heart, mind, and soul—but also a call to oneself.
—Václav Havel, "The Measure of the New Man"	—Robert Coles, *The Call of Service: A Witness to Idealism*

Medical education does not exist to provide students with a way of making money, but to insure the health of the community.

—Paul Farmer, in Tracy Kidder, *Mountains beyond Mountains*

Community Health: The Course

The impetus for launching the Rush Community Service Initiatives Program came from a first-year course in community health I taught in the late 1980s. The primary aim of the course was simply to get the students outside the walls of the academic health center and into the vast cultural diversity of Chicago's neighborhoods and communities. The course was a logistical nightmare. Since the majority of transportation to and from the various sites was by car, and students lived all over the city (a large number in the hip North Side neighborhoods), the scheduling for both the students and the sites willing to accept them was mind-boggling.

When I proposed this course, I was met with mute but evident signs of annoyance; many students saw it as an interference with valuable study time needed to cram for the quarterly basic-science exams. From the medical college administration, the feeling was trepidation that "going into the community" might result in some serious (read: legal) problems. This attitude persisted for quite a while. But since no one was actually willing to stop the course, I stubbornly forged ahead.

Course requirements were simple and straightforward. Small groups of two to five students were assigned to visit on consecutive Tuesdays three different prearranged sites that included neighborhood clinics, public health centers, social service agencies, and a vast array of other community health settings mostly in poor, minority neighborhoods. Two days after these visits, on a Thursday afternoon, a practicing clinician and one other faculty member with a behavioral science, public health, or social medicine orientation facilitated a two-hour small-group discussion with about fifteen students. Prior to the community visit, the students were given a checklist of things to be alert for and gauge—staff morale, quality of services, and client satisfaction as well as signs of poverty and anomie in the community—to guide them in summarizing their experiences. The faculty was also provided a list of questions to help them elicit open responses from the students. A five-page critique on one of the issues that emerged from the community experiences could be submitted for consideration of an honors grade. Otherwise, fulfilling the site visits and discussion sessions resulted in a passing grade. There were no textbooks or assigned readings; this was meant to be purely experiential learning.

The discussion sessions revealed the overwhelming impact of the community experiences on the students. Exposed for the first time in their lives (with a few exceptions) to a vastly different world from the one they were accustomed to, the students rarely refrained from voicing their opinions and feelings about what they saw. At times the exchanges became highly charged. The students in the class represented their own multiculturalism, ranging from third-generation Asian Americans to recent immigrants from Eastern Europe and the Middle East. They talked openly about how they felt with respect to the poor and such ethnic minorities as African Americans and Latinos. For a few, the experiences confronted their prejudices and, on occasion, racist attitudes. About a quarter of the students seemed noncommittal but deeply interested; for at least a third, going into impoverished communities aroused a strong sense of injustice about the huge number of people who are virtually outside the health care system yet housed in the very shadow of one of the largest medical-center complexes in the country. This group expressed an equally strong sense of the need for action to alleviate such inequity. The few Latino and African American students in the class tended to be more restrained in their comments, preferring to observe how their fellow students responded to the site visits. As I went from session to session, I could sense the profound effect these community experiences were having on many of the students. For most of them it was culture shock, pure and simple. It was also a strong indication that even limited exposure to these conditions rekindled the idealism that got so many of them to seek a career in medicine, a theme I return to again and again.

The course ended with each of the discussion groups presenting an oral report of its observations and experiences to a panel of community representatives made up primarily of leaders from grassroots organizations. The students felt uncomfortable about how they might be judged by the community leaders. I found this to be a healthy tension. Although the local community people asked some pointed questions (why do *you* think there are so many black teenage girls with young children and babies?), there wasn't one hostile comment or gesture toward the students. In fact, the community members praised the students for their willingness to come to "their place" to witness their daily struggles.

Community Service: The Plan

At the end of the course, a small group of students came to my office to voice their concern that such experiences were otherwise missing from their formal education. They spoke openly about the fear of losing their motivation for becoming doctors and being caught up, instead, in the competition for grades and esoteric knowledge. They wanted the full complement of knowledge and skills required to become competent doctors, but these community experiences had given them an awareness of the magnitude of difficulties that poor, sick, minority people face on a regular basis, especially those who are uninsured and lack access to quality care. Seeing these disparities in health care for themselves was a revelation. It had tapped some deeply felt concern about their moral obligation as doctors. Most of them came from families and communities that "protected" them from such reality. When I told them that there was no other course in the curriculum offering these kinds of experiences, the students were intent on undertaking some form of community service on their own. I asked them jokingly if they wanted to create their own medical school, and their response was "whatever it takes."

The idea of community service is not new. It became part of the national consciousness in the 1980s. In addition to its intrinsic value, community service became a merit badge for high school graduates seeking acceptance to college. Every personal statement for admission to medical school, with the exception of those from applicants totally engrossed in bench research, includes a detailed account of their voluntary service, much of it in hospitals and nursing homes.

As a way of keeping these community service interests alive, health professional schools instituted a number of programs under the rubric of service-learning. In 1995 the Health Professional Schools in Service to the Nation

(HPSISN) started as a national initiative "to develop, implement, and institutionalize service-learning in health professional education." In 1996 Community-Campus Partnerships for Health (CCPH) was created "to foster partnerships between communities and educational institutions that build on each other's strengths and develop their roles as change agents for improving health professions education, civic responsibility, and the overall health of communities." Yet, from my perspective, these more conventional service-learning experiences have their shortcomings. Hafferty (2000), for example, believes that "for the most part, . . . these types of curricular experiences remain in the control of faculty and administrators, are elective and selected by those who least 'need' them, and thus stand as isolated islands of 'authenticity' in a sea of egoism and entitlement" (30).

Robert Coles (1993), in his highly personal account of his own volunteer work, sees himself as "a witness to idealism." What makes this reflection especially meaningful is his ability—part intuition, part experience, and part knowledge—to capture the relationship between the commitment to service and the satisfaction that comes from "something done, someone reached." The key concept here is "commitment to service." It wasn't required; no one made him do it. In other words, it was an altruistic act and at the heart of his dedication and work that would serve as a model for me in guiding the students.

In my initial discussions with the students, I tried to be pragmatic by pointing out that to establish a viable program that was voluntary and student-run, a number of considerations had to be addressed and certain tasks undertaken prior to starting. We agreed that to be successful the program had to provide continuity of service, be sustainable, and be not simply a onetime event. It should also demonstrate its efficacy through some form of appraisal. Since this was not a research study, evaluation would have to be developed as the program evolved, not the best situation for analysis.

The name Rush Community Service Initiatives Program (RCSIP) emerged from these free-flowing, intense, at times heated, but always exciting discussions. It soon became referred to by the students as "rik sip." I encouraged them to write a thoughtful and lucid statement about what they wanted to achieve. They wrote that their goal was to "create a thriving, self-perpetuating, and sustainable network of community service programs that matched their motivation and commitment with the social and health needs of poor and deprived communities and populations." They devised five obtainable (in their estimation) objectives: (1) develop open and trusting relationships with underserved and disadvantaged communities, (2) provide clinical and social services to those populations based on community need, (3) create a network of service-learning programs, (4) enhance their clinical competence and cultural sensitivity through active community service, and (5) demonstrate that these community partnerships can serve as a mechanism for a collaborative effort between the academic health center and the communities being served. Because they saw in their community health course visits the need for social support, education, counseling, and personal guidance, the students recognized that their focus should not be limited to clinical interventions. In short, it was *service* that really drove them. Keep in mind, these ideas came from them; I simply helped frame them.

Throughout this planning stage, I held a number of meetings at my home. I wanted them to think more deeply about what such an endeavor actually entailed, and the best environment for that was over a beer or glass of wine outside the medical school. I saw my role as helping them to temper their enthusiasm with an awareness of the magnitude of what they were trying to accomplish. I explained that they were literally going against the grain of conventional medical education. Actually, they cherished this notion. They fed on it. It was almost cathartic. It was an avenue for becoming the kind of physician they wanted to be.

Sitting on the floor of my living room, we talked a lot about what it would take to pull this off. In retrospect, the students seemed to have internalized two points that I made. First, drawing on my experiences in the civil rights movement in Mississippi, I told them that they had to "make themselves vulnerable to the community they served." In other words, if they listened closely and didn't try to take over, the community, through its representatives, would lead them to what was needed. They had a hard time grasping this concept initially, but later when they were out in the community (at clinics, community centers, or schools) and had been giving service for a while, they understood what I meant. Second, I reiterated that my job was not to tell them what to do, but, instead, gently prod them to keep them on the right path. I explained to them that I was there as their partner. Moreover, they were the ones responsible for the program's achievement and with that responsibility went overcoming obstacles, solving problems, and addressing unanticipated consequences—the standard issues of any new program.

There were four second-year students who had earlier approached me about their feeling of being isolated from medicine as they had envisioned it and who played pivotal roles in these preliminary days of planning and implementation: Tony Jackson, now an ophthalmologist; Greg Thompson, a general internist; Jenny English, a family doctor; and Peter DeGolia, a geriatrician. The talk was free-flowing and rapid. I remember we used a flow chart, and when a particular concern was identified, one of us wrote it down. As I recall, the list, not necessarily in this order, contained the following: physicians to supervise the students; clearance from the legal office to practice; medicines and supplies; directors to advise; office space; institutional acceptance and recognition; financial support; program protocols; orientation; and last but not least, community partners.

Peter was the recognized leader of the group, not only because he was a former community organizer and was older but also because of his maturity, sensitivity, and integrity. Peter was genuine. When he spoke, everyone listened. Peter was not only the original architect of RCSIP but also the designated spokesman of the group. Most important of all, he was already volunteering at St. Basil's Free People's Clinic in the Englewood neighborhood on Chicago's South Side and was willing to use his credibility as an entrée. This was to be our first clinic venture. His account of the emergence of RCSIP as a progressive student movement serves as the foundation for understanding what these programs meant to all the student participants over the course of more than a decade. He is a very thoughtful person and the depth of his reflections on the origins of RCSIP and the scope of issues to be addressed are instructive:

I chose to attend Rush Medical College after sitting in on a course on social medicine taught by Professor Eckenfels, who was also the assistant dean for academic counseling at that time. I was impressed that there was a course that encouraged medical students to look beyond the biophysical aspects of medicine and get them to understand the impact of a person's culture and social environment on their health. I also wanted to participate in a more interactive and creative method of medical education. The alternative curriculum program was a problem-based educational plan that sought to intertwine basic sciences and clinical training with the case [study] method. As an older student, I knew that I learned best by integrating academic material with life experiences. I expected to be taught not just how to cure diseases, but also to care for people.

Ideally, medicine instills in us the principles of professionalism and its core values. I view the heart and soul of medicine to be caring for people. Throughout my tenure as a medical student at Rush and even before I started medical school, I volunteered at St. Basil's Free People's Clinic. I found that it offered me that critical link between academic training and clinical caring. It afforded me an opportunity to interact in a constructive way with health professionals and people in need of health care.

It wasn't too long after I started medical school that I realized that I had the organizing skills to work with other students who shared my interests to help craft an innovative and comprehensive training program. Nonetheless, I recognized that we could not achieve such a task alone. As suggestions and barriers were raised, we discussed these issues as a team and worked to resolve them.

While we sought to leverage student altruism to care for those less fortunate than ourselves or who had no access to quality medical care, we also learned a great deal about the meaning of collaboration. We learned how to organize meetings and how to clarify thoughts and put concepts into practical application. We wrote articles and developed poster presentations.

In retrospect the Rush Community Service Initiatives Program represented my "most important class." Cultural and social aspects of the human experience interacted with academic medicine in a way that directly impacted my future as a physician. I chose to seek training as a family physician and geriatrician. As a result of this experience I was able to create a community-based outpatient training component in my family medicine residency. I served as a National Health Service Corps physician in the inner city of Cleveland, Ohio, for several years. I also assumed medical director responsibilities of a county-owned nursing facility with multiple problems. Subsequently, I advanced to the position of medical administrator for long-term-care services within one of the largest public health systems in the United States. I remain engaged in medical education and clinical services as director of the Center on Geriatric Medicine at University Hospitals in Cleveland and associate professor of family medicine at Case Western Reserve University School of Medicine.

For Peter, the drive was there from the beginning. He volunteered at St. Basil's before there was a RCSIP. But as RCSIP emerged as a viable entity, his sound judgment, integrity, leadership abilities, and other humanistic attributes emerged as well. He was instrumental in devising ways of addressing the long list of items that had been created. Assignments were divided among the original organizers to be completed as soon as possible. There was no specific order of action to be taken because most efforts took place simultaneously and converged with one goal in mind—making RCSIP operational.

When it came to finding physician-supervisors, the students decided they would only approach faculty members because they wanted to ensure that the medicine they would be practicing was overseen by the most experienced physicians. They put letters in the mailboxes of the attending staff asking for physicians who were willing to supervise them one night a week at St. Basil's. What the recruitment strategy lacked in numbers, it made up for in quality and commitment. Twenty-five physicians, many of whom were well established and had years of experience, responded positively. Dr. William Schwer, head of family medicine, and seven members of his department volunteered. The primary care physicians—family doctors, general internists, and pediatricians—who responded showed they were committed to helping the students. Moreover, since primary care doctors practice ambulatory care outside the academic health center, this was a great opportunity for them to demonstrate how they practiced medicine.

Faculty rank ranged from instructor to professor. Some senior residents also wanted to get involved. Pediatrics was represented by Dr. Richard Belkengren and internal medicine by Drs. Andy Davis and Tom Madden. Referrals were accepted by the Departments of Ophthalmology, Neurology, and Dermatology and the section of cardiology; mammograms and ultrasounds would be given by radiology without charge. Carrie Schlaffer, of preventive medicine, taught the students how to take blood pressures on the basis of the criteria developed by the Joint National Committee on standards for blood pressure measurements. Members of the Behavioral Science Department cooperated as coordinators for psychological interventions. Physicians from the section of infectious diseases kept the students abreast of the latest findings on tuberculosis, sexually transmitted diseases, and AIDS. RCSIP also got help from the Department of Pharmacology in setting up the medication distribution area at St. Basil's. Faculty participation was entirely voluntary and outside the formal system.

This is what Dr. Schwer, family practice chair, said about his initial involvement in RCSIP:

> I am not sure how I became involved in St. Basil's Free People's Clinic at its start. I think I was swept up by the enthusiasm of the students. I remember the first night when all the students came to the original orientation. We must have had at least a hundred students crammed into the rectory. People were sitting everywhere. It was like the sixties when we had sit-in demonstrations against the Vietnam War. The same enthusiasm and commitment was evident everywhere. Each night I spent at St. Basil's was extremely rewarding, and I left feeling good about what we had accomplished but most of all I felt good about myself.

The students, I believe, were able to maintain that sense of service which drove most of them to become physicians. They learned leadership, responsibility, and I am sure came away each night feeling good about themselves.

Several years after St. Basil's ended, a student approached me about helping at CommunityHealth [see chapter 2]. Since I do not speak Spanish and also live on the South Side and [the clinic] is on the North Side, I was initially dubious. Again, the enthusiasm and commitment of the students gave me no choice but to agree to coordinate the physician attendance as I did at St. Basil's. One night just looking at the facility convinced me that I needed to volunteer my time there. Again, when I leave, I have that same sense about myself. I must thank the students for involving me again and look forward to many rewarding years.

In addition to the senior faculty such as Dr. Schwer, there were younger primary care physicians who, under great pressure from their own departments to succeed in their practices as well as their careers, were still willing to give up one to two nights a month to mentor students in an ambulatory care setting that was outside their formal medical training. According to conventional wisdom, this was taboo. Regardless, they loved it. They treated the students as junior colleagues, went over each case carefully, respectfully entertained students' "dumb" questions, introduced social and cultural factors and their influence on the health and well-being of patients, and in the process debunked the myth that primary care is routine medical practice that dulls the inquisitive mind of a potential lifelong learner. The students called it "slow medicine." They learned by slowing down and posing good questions about the patients that resulted in better diagnosis and treatment. Throughout the decade of the 1990s, RCSIP needed to recruit only a few new physicians. There was never a situation—clinical or nonclinical—where faculty did not freely come forward to help.

RCSIP student leaders solicited medications and equipment from various drug company representatives throughout the hospital and made it known that they were looking for equipment that might be put to good use at the clinic.

The students sought help from the Rush legal office. Max Brown, the general counsel for the medical center, was gracious and supportive in all ways. He informed them about the Good Samaritan Act and how it was employed in Illinois. The act states that in any setting (clinic or hospital hallway) where free care is administered, the legal statement that those providing the free care are not culpable must be posted in a place where all those using the service can see it. At St. Basil's the statute was posted in both English and Spanish. Max also hired a part-time law student to help the medical student leaders delineate procedures they could perform that corresponded to the different levels of their training. Under these legal guidelines, the students developed protocols that covered their capabilities at each stage of their formal education.

It was time for me to define my role as well. Since I was already guiding them, I accepted their request to serve as faculty advisor. As a sign of support, my department chair, Dr. James A. Schoenberger, allowed me to oversee RCSIP from my office in preventive medicine. When Dr. Schoenberger retired, his successor, Dr. Henry Black, continued to give the students access to the department as long as they did not interfere with daily operations. Of real significance was the fact that, with the support of the department, I was able to hire Claudia Baier as a full-time assistant director. In addition, we were provided secretarial support that eventually resulted in a full-time position. Claudia had a public health and health education background and was invaluable in helping me with the community service course and related activities. Now it was possible for her to have a well-defined permanent position. From the beginning we were codirectors and partners. In 1991 the RCSIP office was officially established within the Department of Preventive Medicine, conveniently located between the medical school classrooms and the student lounge. It consisted of two modestly equipped offices, with space for a secretary and a student office as well as a storage area. Full access was granted to the department library, meeting rooms, and copy machines. Enthusiasm for these new endeavors seemed to permeate the entire department, helping students to feel welcomed and supported.

But for RCSIP to survive as an acknowledged part of Rush, funding had to be obtained. As soon as she became full time, Claudia took on this responsibility. An initial source of support was the Office of Philanthropy and Communications. Claudia worked primarily with Carol Covington and Patty Shea, who were instrumental in helping to acquire start-up funding.

When it became known that Rush medical students were serving the inner-city poor, this office took note of its public relations potential. This is not to say that the office wasn't fully committed to helping RCSIP succeed in serving poor and disadvantaged communities. In fact, the office was able to get RCSIP its first grant from AT&T a month after Claudia became full time. Although it was not the largest grant RCSIP received ($25,000 a year for two years), it was a start and a good sign that RCSIP wanted to pay its own way rather than be an expense to the medical center. Shortly after the AT&T funding, we received a $300,000 seed grant from the Lloyd A. Fry Foundation. This money was used to support the codirectors' salaries; hire a full-time secretary; and pay for numerous RCSIP undertakings, including materials and supplies, travel expenses to make presentations at professional meetings, needed equipment for the clinics, and models for the health education sessions. During the course of RCSIP's history over the first ten-year period, more than $1.6 million was raised (see appendix A).

The medical college administration was concerned with student safety and distraction from or interference with their formal education. Participants' safety was given utmost importance and stressed at all RCSIP orientation sessions. To address the safety concerns, we developed a protocol with specific guidelines, such as traveling in groups, parking in designated areas, and only visiting the site during specified times (see appendix B). The RCSIP team established its own monitoring system to screen for academic difficulties, relying primarily on an honor system of voluntary disengagement, an excellent example of the core values of trust and honesty. At the end of the first academic year after RCSIP was started, there were no reports of any academic problems among the active participants.

Dr. Larry Goodman, associate dean for medical student programs at that time, quelled any residual concern on the part of some faculty members by giving his full support from the start. Without his willingness to intervene, RCSIP might not have got off the ground. He agreed with my assessment that since the students were adults and RCSIP was being conducted outside scheduled class hours, there was in fact no way we could stop them if we had wanted to. In other words, they could do it with us or without us. Still, we could wash our hands of what they were attempting by announcing that none of the action was approved by Rush.

Dr. Goodman was impressed with how the students had gone about getting RCSIP organized—the faculty recruitment, the meeting with the legal affairs office, the checklist of things that needed to be in place, and obstacles that needed to be overcome. The students took great care to keep him informed of all their undertakings. He was especially concerned about what procedures students at different levels of training would be performing. One function of these clearly stated duties and responsibilities was to make sure that less-qualified student participants were limited in what they could do. I was proud of the students; they had tried hard to anticipate all the obstacles.

For RCSIP to function effectively, an organizational structure was formed to oversee operations. To this end, the students established their own executive and steering committees. The steering committee leaders had responsibility for the operation and maintenance of their particular programs. The executive committee was made up of all the program leaders and focused on the overall direction of RCSIP and maintaining the flow of communication between projects. Claudia was especially effective at overseeing these meetings. An advisory committee consisting of department chairs was also created but would convene only when needed to resolve a problem. In the beginning, the student committees met frequently, but as things got under way, the meetings were scheduled for about once a month, after classes in the preventive medicine conference room, during the evening in an empty classroom, or on Saturday mornings in the hospital cafeteria.

A duty that required concerted effort on the part of the student organizers was familiarizing their classmates with the RCSIP philosophy and its stated aims. First, they had to consider how to introduce RCSIP to the new matriculants at orientation, and, second, students who signed up to participate needed to undergo special training designed to meet the requirements of safety and the objectives of the particular project(s) in which they were to participate. All clinic projects required fundamental training in ambulatory care. A different set of guidelines was created for nonclinical activities. Since the focus there was primarily on education and counseling, specific protocols were designed for each project that included training and implementation components.

Once I received permission from the associate dean and the support of my chairperson to guide the program, I knew that RCSIP was going to become a reality. There was still, however, an overarching concern about operational costs and insurance coverage for patients that might need to be hospitalized. Regarding the latter point, I argued (to anyone who would listen) that since the main purpose of any medical procedure or social service offered by RCSIP was primary health care with an emphasis on disease prevention and health promotion, there was little chance that a wave of uninsured patients would suddenly require hospitalization at Rush. Nevertheless, this worry, just below the surface, did not go away easily. The test of my premise would be what happened once the program was running.

The students had their own anxieties; they particularly feared not being accepted by inner-city communities. They still worried that since most of them were white, privileged, and in the process of becoming physicians, there was no reason why poor blacks or Latinos should trust them. Furthermore, they were medical students, not real doctors, so what did they have to offer? Obviously, they were also concerned about being able to keep up with their studies. To do poorly academically while being active in RCSIP could prove to be a disaster for them and for the program.

There were still some vociferous faculty members who remained skeptical of the value of such "voluntary" community service. For them, students had more important things to do with their time if they wanted to become truly competent physicians; what clinical skills could they possibly offer? It is important to remember that RCSIP started before clinical preceptorships were introduced in the preclinical phase of undergraduate medical education, in which students learn to take histories and physicals in a patient setting.

The tensions generated by this uncertainty cannot be overstated. It always seemed to be just below the surface even after RCSIP was in full swing, and it never seemed to go away completely. As it happened, it became a powerful force for spurring the students on. I came to realize that this kind of stress operated differently from the stress of academic performance. What was at stake in RCSIP was their identity as dedicated health care providers, and it seemed to make them hardier and more committed. As RCSIP evolved and new projects emerged, there was continual reassessment to make sure that no concerns were overlooked. To be prepared to deal with any unexpected results worked as a built-in motivator. The students were totally dedicated to making RCSIP work in a way that would be satisfying for them and for faculty, the administration, and the patients and communities they served. This was not a frivolous notion or a fad; it was at the core of the students' sense of worth. They were afraid that if they lost RCSIP, medicine for them would become primarily instrumental—restricted to the procedures and technical skills that have submerged compassion and empathy.

Rush Community Service Initiatives Program: The Program

When the planning was over and all the components were in place, it was time to make them work. What remained was the biggest challenge of all—community acceptance. Since we had already created a network of community representatives, Claudia and I also took the responsibility for setting up the first community contacts. We sought out local community organizations, clubs, or simply residents—people who could speak for the community. Additionally, we contacted existing agencies, government sponsored and private, but our approach was basically "populist" because, first and foremost, the students wanted to be accepted by the people they were to serve. Although the students had received positive responses from their presentations in the community health course, gaining community acceptance for RCSIP required a great deal of negotiation with community leaders and local boards.

Initially, many local residents were dubious. Even though in theory we had anticipated something like this, it was still a jolt for the students. In general, residents saw us as representatives of the big, private medical center that catered to patients with insurance or money, and, as far as they could tell, in the past Rush had been impervious to the health care needs of the local population that was uninsured. They wanted to know, Why this sudden change of heart? Furthermore, Chicago is notorious for having an abundance of universities and colleges that have preyed on the goodwill of poor urban neighborhoods for research purposes with few positive results for the people who live there.

For those living in the Henry Horner housing project or in the Near West Side community area (almost all African American) and the Pilsen community (Latino), the primary place to go for ambulatory health care in the large West Side medical care complex had been the Fantus Clinic of Stroger (formerly Cook County) Hospital, one of the largest public hospitals in the country.

I counseled the students to view this as a reality check. Given this history, albeit much of it exaggerated, it was understandable that they would be suspicious of a hospital that they believed they had had little or no access to if that hospital suddenly offered some form of service. The situation was further exacerbated by the fact that in the 1970s Rush had overseen the Mile Square Health Center, which was funded by the Office of Economic Opportunity (OEO) as part of President Lyndon B. Johnson's War on Poverty. This free clinic, less than a mile away across the Eisenhower Expressway, provided comprehensive primary care with referrals to Presbyterian–St. Luke's Medical Center, if necessary. When OEO ended, so did the medical center's support. Because of this, there was still lingering resentment among many of the old-timers in the neighborhood.

Another factor that made community people wary was that the students were not actually representing the medical center but were acting on their own with limited official institutional support. This ambiguity remained a source of frustration, and it took a great deal of time and frank discussion to persuade the local residents to let us demonstrate our sincerity and commitment. To put it simply, at first local people tended not to trust us (ironically, we were too connected with the hospital or we weren't connected enough), and so we had to work especially hard to gain their confidence. This double-edged sword of being both independent and representative would haunt us on other occasions. The ambivalence toward the "health care system" provided a tremendous learning experience for the student leaders who went with us to meet community representatives from local organizations. But in the final analysis, it was the students' honesty that became the major factor in the acceptance process. The students displayed a sincere willingness to make themselves vulnerable to the community, and they made it clear that they had physician collaborators to guide them in delivering quality health care. Fortunately for RCSIP, in 1988 the Rush Department of Family Medicine had started a community health clinic in Pilsen, run by Dr. Steven Rothschild. The outstanding care Steve and his staff provided gave Rush a positive face in that nearby community. This advanced the students' case by showing their commitment and ability to serve; like

Dr. Rothschild, they could be a vital link to the academic health center. In this respect, the students actually became goodwill ambassadors for Rush.

Sue Thompson's observations about the early stages of RCSIP are particularly revealing. After graduation, she did her residency in internal medicine at Georgetown University Medical Center, where she started community service programs in the Washington, DC, area. She received numerous awards for her activities, including being selected as one of the outstanding residents of the year by the Association of American Medical Colleges (AAMC). She is now married with two children, practices in central Illinois, and also teaches residents. This is what she has to say:

> I was active in the beginning by helping out with starting and then helping to organize the free clinic project at St. Basil's. I then also helped out on the planning committee as RCSIP developed and evolved into many more service projects.
>
> [RCSIP] was most important in that it helped me to really make a difference. It also helped me to maintain some of the idealism that I came to medical school with. I saw that flame go out in a lot of my classmates who didn't participate in any of the RCSIP projects. I still see it now that I am an academician. Our students and residents become cynical. Those who feel they are making a difference seem to enjoy what they are doing and are better physicians because of their community commitment.
>
> [RCSIP] broadened my experience with the underserved and helped me understand them more as people rather than patients. It helped me to understand medical systems and barriers to access on a more real level. It gave me confidence that I can successfully complete a project, no matter how hard it may seem. It made me realize that no ideas are stupid or too big to achieve.

In the classic sociological study of medical education, *Boys in White: Student Culture in Medical School* (1961), there is a chapter titled "The Fate of Idealism in Medical School." Although this work was written more than forty-five years ago, Becker and his colleagues described the same feelings expressed by Sue, namely, the first thing to go in the effort to survive the rigors of medical training is one's idealism, to be replaced by a practical assessment of what it is important to know in order to survive and hopefully achieve academic success. RCSIP kept Sue's idealism alive. But now as an academic, she tries not only to hang on to her idealism but also to instill it in her students and residents who have already become cynical. The message she wants to share is that idealism doesn't detract from competence. It's quite an effort, but her idealism is her sustenance and, as manifested in her attitude toward her patients, is a source of personal satisfaction. I saw the full force of that idealism come to fruition in her commitment to make RCSIP a reality, especially in the St. Basil's prenatal clinic (discussed in chapter 2).

As codirectors of the program, Claudia Baier and I were involved in all phases of RCSIP's implementation. We worked with the students, faculty, medical center administration, Office of Philanthropy and Communications on an ongoing basis. We also spent a great deal of time outside the medical center meeting community representatives. In all these endeavors, numerous meetings were set up, moderated, and recorded. Assignments were made. Results were reported. Obstacles were identified. Unforeseen problems were addressed. The dynamic continued at a fast pace.

Just prior to starting, I took great care to clarify that it is impossible to administer truly comprehensive health care to the poor and disadvantaged through voluntary community service programs. The students needed to know that they could not meet the health care needs of the homeless with one or two nights a week at a free clinic. Furthermore, I warned them that naysayers would criticize their efforts because of that. Lack of adequate, accessible, and quality health care is a problem for our society and characterizes the present crisis in medicine. The same logic applies to the tutoring and counseling endeavors. Does this mean that RCSIP efforts are meaningless? Of course not. They do provide some needed care and support to people who have no other sources. I pointed out that to some degree these endeavors extended life and alleviated suffering.

The greatest potential of what RCSIP has to offer lies in its exposing future doctors to what it is like to be homeless, poor, black, Latino, or a member of another minority group caught in these difficult conditions. Since before you can reform, you have to have some basis of understanding, this new awareness served to foster the participants' pledge as dedicated change agents. This is what Howard Gardner and his cognitive development and "good works" team at Harvard call the development of an enduring commitment to service work (Gardner, Csikszentmihalyi, and Damon 2001). That is the real payoff. Because doctors have duties and responsibilities to society, the seed is planted and the commitment is reinforced. It is building reform one citizen doctor at a time.

I want to emphasize again that as codirectors of RCSIP Claudia and I never told the students what to do, how to run things, or who should be in charge. As RCSIP advisors and student confidants, we were asked to help directly in areas where we had special expertise such as project organization, program evaluation, and health education. Otherwise, we mostly raised questions and provided feedback. If there was a conflict or dilemma and our advice was sought, we responded with "The final decision rests with you." We intervened independently only when an issue of safety, malpractice, or potential conflict was involved. As one student put it, the directors' job was to "gently nudge us to make sure we were doing the right thing."

From the start, we became trusted teachers and friends for the most activist students. Claudia spent many hours, almost daily, listening to the students talk about their concerns and aspirations. The students used their time with us as a forum for reflection. Rapport developed naturally. They were not shy about expressing their concerns about their own motivation, the ethical dilemmas surrounding the practice of medicine, their disappointments, and in short their quest for meaning as future doctors dedicated to the call of service. We were also able to oversee and articulate RCSIP as a totality that enhanced the learning and development progression. We raised this perspective frequently in discussions about specific projects. Our aim was to get the students to recognize that they were part of something bigger, which, in turn, got them to think more inclusively. We found that this systems approach yielded a notion of social responsibility as well as individual rights. RCSIP was the nexus of a bond that holds individuals together.

To capture the full measure of RCSIP requires an operational framework capable of taking into account its heuristic nature. In other words, because RCSIP was dynamic and evolving, it required constant attention. Like all aspects of the program, outcomes are evolving. To confront this process squarely required a constant critical examination of how things were going. Under our guidance, this was the primary function of the various committees the students had organized.

As participant-observer, I was able to get the full picture of what constitutes RCSIP as it evolved. I relied on observations, reflections, narratives, and other methods used by anthropologists and sociologists to get at the feeling and meaning of RCSIP for *all* its participants. There is a general skepticism about narratives and anecdotes in medical education. It is assumed that they detract from the logical and deductive reasoning of science. I concur with Rita Charon (1993), a general internist who teaches writing and interviewing skills to medical students and residents, who has stated, "Narrative knowledge . . . concerns motivations and the consequence of human actions" (149). For me, this is what service-learning is all about.

From the inception of RCSIP, I stressed that the students write up their experiences. I worked with the students to help them produce more scholarly papers. The students also gave presentations at local and national meetings. Again, the emphasis was on quality and substance. For approximately a five-year period RCSIP students played a major role in the American Medical Students Association and made presentations at its national meetings on the value of RCSIP as a student-run community service program or how a particular project functioned. Accompanied by RCSIP student representatives, Claudia and I gave a number of presentations at the AAMC. We also conducted a study group for those interested in starting their own programs. As part of the fund-raising process, we had the good fortune to become members of the Health of the Public (HOP), which was financed by the Pew Charitable Trust and the Robert Wood Johnson Foundation in collaboration with the Rockefeller Foundation. The HOP initiative (composed of thirty-three academic health centers at the time Rush joined) was dedicated to advancing a population perspective through community relationships, curricular reform, and collaboration among the health professions.

By becoming members of this vital and innovative group, we were able to meet each year with our new colleagues, both academic and community based, at one of the sites where we would discuss common problems, share experiences, and visit local programs. We were able to develop important and deeply rewarding friendships with a number of outstanding health professionals and community leaders. During our second year in HOP, we served as the host institution. Our colleagues had an opportunity to visit many of our sites, meet our community partners, and celebrate our achievements with a Chicago blues band at the banquet on the final night. These relationships continue to this day, and we were proud of being able to contribute to a clearinghouse of program outcomes and lessons learned—a valuable resource for anyone interested in community health through the creation of community partnerships.

By way of summary, in our role as program directors Claudia and I were able to witness the maturation, learning, and development of a dedicated group of future physicians. From the first consideration, we were able to follow the evolution of RCSIP in great detail. The vividness of what RCSIP meant to the participants comes from listening to the students' accounts of their personal experiences, talking to community people about their impressions of the students' involvement, hearing from the faculty who guided them, observing the impact of student participation on their clients/patients and the communities they serve, and generally reflecting on what these community service activities meant to them and the people they helped. The remainder of the book is dedicated to telling the rest of the RCSIP story and its implication for social reform.

Chapter 2

Clinics Serving the Poor and Homeless

Many people feel empty and don't know why they feel empty. The reason is we are social animals and we must live and interact and work together in community to become fulfilled.

—Robert N. Bellah, Richard Madsen, William M. Sullivan, Ann Swidler, and Steven M. Tipton, *Habits of the Heart: Individualism and Commitment in American Life*

We all discovered that in our academic centers it's hard to become passionate about something that you don't see or experience personally. All of us ended up choosing careers that were very different from what we had originally intended. What made us change? Well it wasn't our formal training. It was real life experiences in the community that transformed us.

—Arthur Kaufman, interview in *Education for Health*

Although the four clinics serving the poor and homeless shared the common theme of learning from giving service to the underserved and disadvantaged, each one had its own pattern of what these experiences meant to the RCSIP participants and the people they served. The different geographic areas, the unique history of each community, the broad sociocultural variations, and the social order of each clinic or shelter provided settings in which an understanding of the human element of giving care went far beyond simply learning medical procedures and technical skills. In what follows I try to capture the essence of what these experiences meant to all those who were involved in volunteering their service.

St. Basil's Free People's Clinic

Chicago grew at a startling pace early in the twentieth century. In 1920 the population of the Englewood community was more than 85,000; one-fifth were immigrants, mostly from Sweden, Ireland, and Germany. The neighborhood had a hospital (St. Bernard's), a major shopping center, and the Becker-Ryan building, which became the main plant for Sears, Roebuck, and Company. By 1940 there were more than 150,000 residents living in Englewood. In 1949, when a group of blacks attended a union gathering at the home of a Jewish resident, a rumor circulated that the home was being sold to a black family. More than ten thousand people staged demonstrations against "blacks and Jews, Communists, and University of Chicago meddlers."[1]

In 1950 the second great migration from Mississippi to Chicago began. Cotton picking was being mechanized and there was work in the big city on Lake Michigan. As blacks moved into Englewood, white flight began. A geographical factor of major significance was the construction of the Dan Ryan Expressway, which many believed was intended as a physical barrier to keep blacks in southwest communities such as Englewood. In 1960 the population was almost 70 percent black; by 1970, it was 96 percent.

In 1991, the year that RCSIP started at St. Basil's, the total population was around 48,500, of which more than 99 percent was black. Median income was $13,243. More than half the population under sixty-five was on welfare. More than 88 percent of the births in 1994 were by mothers who were not married; 55 percent of those mothers were under twenty-four years of age. Lead screening showed an elevated rate of 57.6 percent. The third-leading cause of death, after heart disease and stroke, was homicide.[2]

The drive to St. Basil's from Rush is south down Ashland to Garfield, a divided boulevard, with parkland and large trees in its broad center, that runs from Washington Park west. In its heyday, large handsome gray-stone townhouses lined the street; now most of them have been subdivided into many small apartments and need major repair. Although they still looked good on the outside because of their stylish quarry-stone, early 1900s facades, the typical interior revealed peeling lead paint, poor plumbing, faulty wiring, and a shortage of bathrooms. The side streets contained vacant lots and six-flat apartment buildings that were falling apart; 43 percent of the residents lived below the poverty line. During the decade of the 1990s, seven hundred murders occurred.

St. Basil's Free People's Clinic was started in 1981 by Dr. Eric Kast, an internist at Michael Reese Hospital. It is the oldest free clinic in Chicago and has remained one of the few providers of health care in the Englewood community since its inception. Dr. Kast was a devout Catholic convert who believed that true Christian charity was based on altruism and helping the poor. His golden rule was that anyone who sought care at St. Basil's would never have to pay for anything. This philosophy permeated the entire atmosphere of St. Basil's. When Rush students began participating, they were completely taken by it. They were quick to notice the vast difference between what they saw at St. Basil's and the expensive technology at the academic health center and the concerns about cost containment that seemed to be a priority in every procedure from drawing blood to doing a CT scan. Giving health care without charging for it was a totally new concept. The closest thing to paying was a can left at the admissions desk so people who wanted to could leave a donation. One subzero winter evening a homeless man wandered into the clinic, warmed himself for a little while, and then took the one dollar bill and change that was in the can and left. No one even thought to stop him.

The clinic was located in the basement of the old school rectory, which had been closed for twenty years. The building was more than seventy-five years old, and the basement, which was built for storage and housing the boiler, was dark but clean and well kept. When there was a heavy rainfall or the snow started melting, the basement could flood. The floors were far from level because the building had continued to settle since it was first built. There was a small office for the clinic director. A desk, table, and chair served as the reception area. Old church pews from the beautiful Byzantine-style church next door, which had been closed because it was too costly to heat and repair, served as seating for the waiting room. (Sunday mass was held in an auditorium near the school.) The largest room, next to where the boiler was located, served as a quite well equipped dental office, where a small group of committed dentists volunteered their services every night the clinic was open. Four small offices had been converted to examination rooms, providing a little privacy for the doctor seeing a patient. Sinks had been installed, and exam tables and other equipment had been donated by Michael Reese, one of the most prominent hospitals in Chicago at the time that St. Basil's Free People's Clinic was started.

Most of the original physicians who volunteered came from Michael Reese as well. The two Dr. Shapiro brothers, also from Michael Reese, were influential in supporting the idea of having Rush students and doctors join the volunteer medical staff. The majority of patients reflected the demographics of Englewood, but, beginning in the early 1990s, a number of Latinos, mostly Mexican, who live south of Garfield Boulevard, began using St. Basil's as their primary source of health care.

Since Peter DeGolia had already established himself as an able and responsible volunteer at St. Basil's, the group decided to approach the clinic's governing body with the prospect of starting a general medicine clinic to coincide with the care that was already being provided. Making our proposal for such a clinic at St. Basil's a reality required a great deal of planning and preparation on the part of the original group of four, because, in addition to its significance for ambulatory care prospects, it would set the precedent for the establishment of future clinic programs. It was the litmus test. Before RCSIP's general medicine clinic at St. Basil's could become a reality, the students had to be approved by the clinic board. For most of them this was their first encounter with community representatives in a formal setting.

Because Peter was already familiar with the workings of St. Basil's, he was instrumental in arranging the meeting. The students were anxious about how they would be received, but Peter set the right tone. Since it was their first community-based meeting, I attended to make sure the board understood Rush's role in the negotiations. Laura Jones, the executive director of the clinic and the person the students and their physician mentors would be working with, was also present. Peter made our case very succinctly, placing particular emphasis on developing a partnership. I added that such partnerships were a primary goal of the Department of Preventive Medicine. I served chiefly as moral support, while Peter and his student colleagues made the following points: Since we had recruited a number of competent physicians, including the chair of family medicine, to deliver quality health care, a general medicine clinic sponsored by Rush faculty and students could give one additional night each week of medical services to the Englewood community. Moreover, student participants would be carefully supervised by the volunteer physicians, and, in addition, they had access to valuable resources such as referrals for diagnostic tests, free medications, and donated laboratory equipment such as a microscope and examination tables for starters. The St. Basil's Free People's Clinic Board was quite impressed and, with the approval of the clinic director, accepted our proposal for a general medicine clinic on Tuesday evenings.

Prior to seeing patients the students and their physician mentors had to be acclimated to the way the clinic worked. Laura Jones conducted an orientation session for both students and doctors at St. Basil's on a Saturday morning when no patients were around. The orientation was followed by a series of evenings of direct observation while the clinic was in service. In conjunction with their acclimation to St. Basil's, the faculty mentors conducted their own orientation for the students. Fundamental techniques such as taking vital signs and giving injections had to be taught to the preclinical students. At that time medical students did not normally encounter "real" patients until their third year. A special-skills night was established in which the third- and fourth-year (M3, M4) students, under the guidance of their physician mentors, taught the newcomers. The students teaching students was a big hit. Claudia and I spent time preparing them to engage family members in the waiting area and to explain their role as students in conjunction with that of their physician teachers.

Students worked in teams led by M3 and M4 students, who followed panels of patients, while M1 and M2 students interacted with patients prior to their examination and did triage, all under physician supervision. This arrangement facilitated "vertical integration" by not only allowing students to work as a team but also enabling them to move from one stage of responsibility to the next as their knowledge and skills grew. Since the students had attracted supervising physicians mostly from primary care, these doctors were their first contact with the actual practice of medicine. They made excellent mentors to the students, especially since they were not evaluating or grading them. The students were treated as junior colleagues.

Furthermore, the primary care doctors worked in concert—what the students referred to as "horizontal integration"—giving them an opportunity to see the benefits of a cooperative patient care team. Open discussions or teaching sessions gave the student participants a feeling about the patient as a person. Those students who had been talking to the families added the sociocultural dimension to the situation. Some common statements were frequently heard: "My husband was laid off and can't afford his blood pressure pills." "I know Mama's sugar is high but we don't have anything else to eat." "The kids always seem to have the flu, maybe because three of them sleep in one bed." The students learned that the diagnoses—mostly respiratory infections, hypertension, and diabetes—were related not only to physical health but also social well-being.

Once the clinic became a reality in the winter quarter of 1991, a throng of students wanted to participate. A waiting list was created on a first-come-first-served basis. It became apparent that a mechanism was needed to handle the flow of students who wanted in on the action. New participants had to be oriented about how the clinic functioned and the list of procedures that were performed. Prior to starting, there was also an orientation at the clinic on a Saturday. All these tasks had to be organized in terms of policy and procedures. Under the guidance of the original leaders, a group of students stepped forward to take charge. On the basis of their initial willingness to accept responsibility, these students began the process of managing and maintaining RCSIP, a process that was essential to its existence (Eckenfels 2000a). In a short time, the general medicine clinic expanded from one day to two days a week; it operated about forty weeks a year and accounted for about five hundred patient contacts annually over the eight years of its existence. It was not unusual to see as many as fifteen patients in one evening; on those occasions the clinic sometimes remained open until midnight.

The Rush Prenatal Program at St. Basil's Free People's Clinic was the brainchild of Sue Thompson and Michelle Bardack, M2 students at that time. On the basis of their experiences, they became concerned about the lack of adequate prenatal and gynecological care for women who were being seen in the general medicine clinic.

In the Englewood community in 1994, the infant and neonatal mortality rates were 41 and 11 per thousand births, respectively. By comparison, the African American infant mortality for Chicago was 18.8 in 1994 and, more recently, 13.6 for the United States in 2003.[3] The social and personal problems that pregnant women brought to the clinic bothered Sue and Michelle a great deal. They also saw the situation as a microcosm of the lack of primary care physicians interested in women's health issues in ambulatory care settings, especially in the inner city. The program they proposed to the St. Basil's board was to address the situation by (1) delivering comprehensive prenatal care to pregnant women through the clinic; (2) providing an environment in which medical students learn, through experience, to be humane, culturally sensitive, and clinically competent in treating the health needs of all female patients; and (3) creating an experience that reinforced the students' interest in practicing community-oriented maternal and child care. Because of the success of the RCSIP general medicine clinic at St. Basil's, the board wholeheartedly accepted the prenatal program proposal.

At the prenatal care clinic over a three-year period, twenty-four medical students, working in teams supervised by Elizabeth Nye, MD, who came from the Department of Obstetrics and Gynecology at Rush and had previous volunteer experience in India, maintained continuity of care by monitoring expectant mothers from pregnancy through delivery and beyond. All participants in the program—students, faculty, patients, and families—were followed to determine the quality of the care delivered. Moreover, the students and their mentors wanted to show that a partnership between an academic medical center and a neighborhood clinic was not only feasible but also cost effective and socially responsible.

The student teams explained to the pregnant women their role as student physicians, produced the histories and performed the physicals, presented the findings to the physicians, and actively participated in maximizing the patients' understanding of their condition. The students also learned how to perform a Pap test. Special diagnostic equipment was purchased and donated to facilitate the care offered at the clinic. Whenever possible, analyses of these tests were completed by the students. When patients needed additional assessments, such as a sonogram, the students arranged for these tests to be conducted at Rush and, whenever possible, attended the procedure. The Department of Obstetrics and Gynecology at Rush provided these tests without cost to the patients. The students played a vital role as patient advocates steering the women through the system. This involved keeping in touch with their patients by phone or mail, helping them obtain public aid and WIC (Women, Infants, and Children) forms, and scheduling appointments at the medical center. As the time of birth approached, the mothers knew they would be met by the student advocates in the maternity area of the hospital. This was to be a showcase model for Rush and the community.

During the two and a half years in which the prenatal clinic was functioning, sixty-five deliveries, all resulting in healthy mothers and infants, took place at Rush–Presbyterian–St. Luke's Medical Center. The medical center provided twenty-four free deliveries a year, absorbed the cost of all laboratory work not covered by other sources, and provided taxi vouchers for the patients to use at delivery time. The mothers ranged in age from fifteen to twenty-seven years, with a mean age of around seventeen. Two-thirds were Latino, the rest African American, and about half were single parents. The program ended when state-sponsored prenatal care became available to the uninsured.

The strong relationships that developed between the expectant mother and the student teams contributed immensely to the mother's health and sense of well-being. During the course of the prenatal care, the medical students observed a growing sense of self-worth on the part of the expectant mothers, who became more cooperative, healthy, and adherent patients. The program provided comprehensive prenatal care that prevented expensive neonatal care. The two students who started the clinic, Bardack and Thompson (1992), received the Secretary of Health and Human Services Award for Innovation in Health Promotion and Disease Prevention.

To gain insight into the significance of the prenatal clinic for all the participants, Michelle took an individual research course with me as a senior elective. She was able to interview fifteen of the thirty patients enrolled in the clinic at that time and eleven of the thirteen students who were administering the prenatal care. Fourteen of the fifteen mothers interviewed rated the quality of care excellent, and many commented that it was the best they had ever received. On a scale of items, they consistently rated the students as personable, sensitive, knowledgeable, and caring. Five of the student respondents said that if their only experience in obstetrics had been on the floors of the medical center, they never would have gone into the field. In fact, six of the eleven students (all women) made family practice their career choice with an emphasis on maternal and child care (Eckenfels 2000a).

Students had some strong comments about their experiences at the clinic: "I realized I wanted to become, and could become, an independent family practitioner with an active obstetrical practice, so I am looking into family practice residencies that offer a strong Ob experience." Sometimes the experience was transformative: "The clinic experience was extremely important to my residency decision, as I quickly learned that doing Ob outside the tertiary care center was indeed very different. It was a great experience to see community Ob (I loved it), whereas I did not get the same feeling about it during my hospital rotation." Moreover, the experience gave the students a true sense of the direction they wanted for their lives: "Usually in my hospital clerkships I learned what kind of doctor I do not want to be; at St. Basil's I was able to learn what kind of doctor I wanted to be—it solidified my ideas to look for a primary care residency." Most of all, the students learned to enjoy their work: "It was a great experience to see community Ob; I loved it, whereas my hospital clerkship almost turned me off."

All the student respondents felt that the experience was highly positive and beneficial. They indicated that they "didn't get exposed to a continuity care experience in school or to such a level of responsibility." As one student put it, the clinic "was unlike any other experience I had in medical school; learning to relate to people of other cultures and backgrounds was as important as the academic experience." Immersion proved to have a powerful effect: "This hands-on experience exposed me to a whole different perspective on health care issues—those outside the hospital. I found myself and my patient sometimes overwhelmed when trying to solve some of the social problems my patient faced."

The students also listed many of the "human problems" they were exposed to: "I picked [the patient] up at her house, and for the first time saw how she lived—with her grandmother and multiple relatives. There was very little heat in the middle of the winter, in a very small apartment, and with little furniture and one bed for a family of four." An awareness of social strata grew in this setting: "For the first time I became aware of the existence of the working poor; I never would have gotten such a sense of community had I remained at the tertiary care hospital for four years; the experience reminded me of the reasons I came to medical school—for service to the community and to develop relationships that help people improve their lives."

What we find in the students' responses is their open and honest acknowledgment of what they were experiencing. You cannot help feeling that the students are talking about what really matters to them currently and as future doctors. In the formal, academic setting, you would not get these kinds of reactions because they would be considered unprofessional with respect to the way physicians in training are taught to think, see, and speak, that is, the way medicine constructs its objects (Good 1994). This is one of the beautiful spin-offs of voluntary service: participants feel free to express such feelings as compassion and empathy. Their actions enhance their sense of purpose. Furthermore, it takes place in a background of responsibility not only to the patient but also to the community where the patient resides. The students weren't satisfied with just delivering the baby; they wanted to see it survive, thrive, and grow into healthy childhood, adolescence, and a full life. They wanted to see the mother in the same context. For those who originally were considering a career in obstetrics and gynecology, family medicine became the best avenue for treating women's health issues.

What the students obtained—practically, intellectually, and emotionally—at St. Basil's was quite remarkable. They had created a health care experience that resonated with their dedication and allowed them to feel confident about why they wanted to become doctors. Trish, currently a family physician with a faculty appointment who sits on a national award committee for excellence in family medicine, was a star throughout medical school. She was essentially "adopted" by family practice and at graduation received the Pisicano Award from the Society of Teachers of Family Medicine. She also spent a lot of time with Claudia reflecting on her RCSIP experiences as they related to her career choice. Her comments are brief but to the point:

> I was very active early on, went to St. Basil's monthly, then became the head of organizing the pharmacy, got drugs from the drug reps, developed a protocol for dispensing the drugs, and the like. I became chairperson of the primary care committee [of RCSIP] and was very involved all four years.
>
> The most valuable part was helping people who really need it, being involved in a true education process: point-of-care education and what we called slow medicine. I learned that good health care required a partnership between the patient and the doctors. It was also so wonderful to interact with positive and wonderful practicing family physicians while still in medical school. It gave more meaning to what we were learning in class.
>
> For me, the most important aspect was [having] involved doctors become my mentors. These experiences focused my interest to family medicine and community health, which is what I currently practice.

Volunteering at St. Basil's was for Trish the perfect path to a career as a family doctor who is medically skilled and socially conscious. The description of having a chance to relate to the patient holistically with a physician mentor who included the social and psychological as well as the biological side of the person's medical problem was expressed again and again by the students. Here was that extra dimension missing from the strictly didactic approach in the clinical concepts and skills course that, in those days, was taught prior to starting clerkship rotations.

Geeta Maker is also a family doctor, married to a physician (a classmate), and has two children. She graduated first in her class at Rush. Since she excelled in every discipline, some department chairs and members of the dean's office were somewhat taken aback when she chose a residency in family practice at a local community hospital. Geeta's motivation and commitments are made clear in her narrative:

I was involved in St. Basil's Free People's Clinic from 1995 to 1998 as a volunteer and a steering committee member. I volunteered every other week for an evening or two, and went to monthly meetings. At the time it was a place where I could put myself to the work of doctoring, a practice I had come to know through my prior international health work in India. During the didactic years in medical school, learning the fundamentals of science was exciting only insofar as it dealt with the future promise of actually listening to, talking to, and touching real people. St. Basil's gave me the chance to be the doctor that I knew I was already, before I had even "learned" to be one in the practical sense. There was a sense of reality and grit to the place, whereas [in conventional training] you only saw patients in the grand halls of academic institutions like Rush.

I didn't come to St. Basil's to get ahead in my clinical practice. I don't think anyone who was active in RCSIP did. That was an unexpected reward. We had a strong sense of social justice. To balance out the inequalities of the health care system, one had to provide care to those who didn't have access. This is a disease of our system that is still nowhere close to being cured and that, even then, when I didn't understand its full extent, I felt needed to be tackled. I think that my experience in RCSIP, in working with like-minded people, in taking our limited free time and donating it to the causes of the poor, only prepared me better for what I hope will be a lifetime of commitment to the underserved. At St. Basil's I saw the underbelly of inner-city life—the homeless and the cold, the alcoholics, drug users, neglected elderly—and that experience brought out so much in me. I felt so much pain, sadness, compassion, anger that ultimately fueled me to devote to a practice where these people would be the recipients of any care I could provide. After medical school I chose a family practice residency in Chicago near one of the poorest communities and worked at a clinic that catered to the needs of the poor and uninsured. There I met even more kindred spirits, mentors, and patients that fed my desire to stay in this sector.

There is a very political nature to being a doctor, whether you want it or not. You make decisions every day about whom you will treat, and how you will treat them, with medications or alternative remedies or interventions. This involves your medical knowledge, yes, but it also involves your conscience, your values, your knowledge about cultural beliefs, about drug prices in pharmacies and street value of the same drugs, your feelings about the poor, in general. You can change people's lives by taking an interest in them, their health, and their struggles. You can stand alongside them as their doctor and try to navigate them to better health and maybe a better place than the one they are in. And by doing that you are making the statement that everyone should have the right to health care, regardless of their station in life. That's what RCSIP was about for me.

I now work as a family physician in Oxnard, California, caring for mostly the Mexican migrant workers who pick fruit in the fields here. I focus mainly on maternal and child health, and providing prenatal care for high-risk pregnancies. Our clinic has resources that enroll people in WIC programs, family-planning insurance programs, MediCal, and free medications. It is the right place for me, and this is the right profession. RCSIP was basically my "Intro to Medicine 101. P.S. Welcome to the rest of your life."

I also asked Michelle Bardack, a family physician who has just returned to New Mexico where she had previously practiced at the clinic in Shiprock, to give her general impressions. As mentioned above, she was a compatriot of Sue Thompson's in starting the prenatal clinic. They were both in the problem-based preclinical curriculum and early activists in RCSIP. She is married and has three children. She offers these humanistic insights:

[As a participant in RCSIP] I learned about the real day-to-day problems that patients face, from inadequate housing to homelessness. I came face to face with the huge problems of the under- and uninsured in the U.S. I saw how much difference a good pair of shoes could make to someone's overall health. Working with a homeless diabetic who won't give a damn about his insulin dose if he doesn't first know where his next meal is coming from. This tension between the doctor's agenda and the patient's would not have been apparent to me if I had met the same patients . . . in a sterile hospital room.

I was introduced to the field of public health—scientifically, socially, and statistically. How to formulate a research question. How to investigate. How to crunch numbers. I learned how to write and rewrite proposals and papers, and give presentations. I became skilled in public speaking, in assuming an administrative role.

Perhaps most enjoyable for me, I became fascinated by the extra challenges faced in cross-cultural medicine, how so much more exists besides a language barrier. The anthropology part of medicine was an entirely new field for me. I loved learning about patients' non-Westernized beliefs and understanding of illness. I tried to work cooperatively with them to find an agreeable treatment plan. Much of this would not have happened had I not been involved in RCSIP.

[RCSIP] influenced me greatly by introducing me to what was to become my passion and joy in medicine—teaching students and residents to not lose sight of their desire to provide care in communities of need [and] realizing the importance of the individual patient but also how that fits into community and public health measures.

These programs provided the foundation—the problem-solving skills, the keen observant eye, and the heart—that I have built upon over the years to become the physician I am today. I learned so much more in the "actual classroom," that is, the clinic, than I ever would have in the lecture hall. In fact, it was these real live patients that I was responsible for that made me hit the books to learn about their health problems and find ways to treat them. For me, this active, independent learning was so much more satisfying than the rote, more passive [process of the] traditional medical school.

There was an unfortunate ending to the partnership between St. Basil's and RCSIP, but it too served as an important lesson for all of us. I attended a meeting of the new board in the fall of 1996. While I was reporting about some of RCSIP's accomplishments over the past year—a fund-raiser, an increase in the number and type of free drugs in conjunction with a reorganization of the pharmacy, equipment donated, and the like—a new board member began to attack Rush as a wealthy institution using St. Basil's Free People's Clinic patients as a source of training for their students, who, after graduation, would go into specialties, make a lot of money, and never serve the poor or people of color again.

I was taken completely off guard. I explained that RCSIP was not Rush per se, but a group of students and physicians who volunteered for the same reasons other health professionals volunteered—to serve those without care. The board member's response was that Rush should be paying St. Basil's for allowing the clinic to be used as a teaching experience. In short, he implied that we were using the patients for our own ends. He had touched a raw nerve at the heart of the clinic, the "purity" of St. Basil's bequeathed by Eric Kast's personal philosophy and medical ethic: free care for the poor. In principle, anything outside that was not in keeping with that basic belief.

I emphasized that the very fact that the service comes from the students and their doctor mentors, independent of the institution, made it voluntary. I pointed out that we were striving to reintroduce the core values that have been lost in medical education. This was to be the start of establishing a true relationship between community clinics and Rush. But it only made things worse. I finished my response with the fact that even if I wanted to (and I didn't) there was no way I could get the academic health center to pay for clinic functions; the notion that we should be paying for each patient encounter enraged me. I was very angry and they knew it. Our contribution to the clinic was too important to me and I lost my cool. I left while the discussion continued. A few days later I received a letter that our relationship was over.

The students were devastated, especially the seniors who had devoted their entire community service efforts to St. Basil's. I took responsibility for ending the relationship, and we spent quite a bit of time dissecting the situation. The original architects of the general medicine and obstetrics and gynecology clinics had graduated, but the current group was aware that St. Basil's was the catalyst for all later RCSIP patient care activities. It was more than the medical services; it was the organization—the procedures, the assignments, the communication with community residents, the physician mentors and fellow classmates, and the leadership that arose from leading by doing. In our discussions, I reminded them that there had always been a sense that regardless of how much we were doing we were still outsiders who, despite our best intentions, were seen as tangential to the true spirit of St. Basil's. I recalled that I was chastised for not asking St. Basil's permission, when I referred to the RCSIP clinics in the first talk I gave about community service, which was later published in a volume by the Association of Academic Health Centers (Eckenfels 1993).

Claudia and I went over all the implications of this event with the students. The lessons learned focused on a series of questions: What does a community need? Who speaks for the community? How does a neighborhood clinic meet those needs? And what is its mission? Tough questions not easily answered, but important in reflection. These are questions and perspectives that these students will take with them through their medical careers.

A brief postscript: Recently I happened to meet a physician who is currently volunteering at St. Basil's. Of course, I had never lost my fondness for the clinic. As we talked he told me that he knew all about RCSIP's liaison with St. Basil's. He said there was still a strong belief among some people (he didn't say who) that we had experimented on the patients. "How?" I asked in disbelief. "Well," he said, "the fact that the two students who started the prenatal clinic had written a paper that won a Secretary of Health and Human Services award in the medical school category showed that they had used the program for their own purposes."

Regardless of how sensitive you think you are being, you can still alienate those who see you as an outsider. It is impossible to avoid this. But you can't despair; to learn and to act on what we have learned—that is how we grow and develop. This was the essence of what I tried to get across to those students who had been so deeply invested in St. Basil's. Ironically, the same physician also told me that the particular instigator of the battle against Rush had been removed from the board. Moreover, he told me that he personally felt that RCSIP's participation would be welcomed if they wanted to return. I told him to call the office that was now overseeing the program.

Pilsen Homeless Services

The fastest-growing ethnic group in Chicago according to the 2000 census is Latino, numbering more than 754,000 individuals, or about 26 percent of the total population. There were about 530,000 Mexican Americans, 18 percent of the city's population. Pilsen and Little Village make up the largest Mexican American community in the Midwest and nationally come in second only to East Los Angeles.[4] Pilsen is the older and more established of the two, with a flourishing commercial area consisting of a museum and restaurants and other businesses located along Eighteenth Street. The music and festive spirit give visitors to the neighborhood the feeling of "Old Mexico." Pilsen is part of the Near West Side, one of the seventy-seven community areas designated by the city. In the late nineteenth century Pilsen was inhabited by Czech immigrants who named the community after the home of their famous beer. Along with Bohemians and Poles, these descendants of Eastern Europe were part of a vast movement to the suburbs in the late 1950s.

Little Village has a more industrial character than Pilsen has. Although prewar frame houses and brick two-flats line the streets, some small factories are found on Thirty-first Street and abandoned train tracks crisscross the neighborhood. Before the large migration of Mexicans in the 1950s, the community, located in South Lawndale, was the home of Italians, Polish, Lithuanians, and Croatians. Today it is also the home of Alivio Medical Center, a grassroots community health care facility that has been directed by Carmen Velasquez since its inception in 1989. Alivio is a full-service, not-for-profit community health center with more than sixteen thousand patient visits annually and approved by the Joint Commissions on Accredited Health Organizations.

The number of residents living in the two communities listed in the 2000 census is around 127,000; 86 percent are primarily Mexican American. These figures do not include the many "undocumented" immigrants who have come to Chicago and its environs looking for work. The more stable population can best be characterized as working class, the majority engaged in the labor and service sectors, with a good proportion classified as the working poor. They are very young, 45 percent being under age thirty-five, with many children. The birthrate is high, but so is the infant mortality rate. Since this Mexican enclave is actually part of two of the seventy-seven community areas, there are no separate vital statistics available for the two neighborhoods. Nonetheless, there are certain observable sociodemographic factors that help describe the area. For example, the majority of the population are devout Catholics with strong family ties both in Chicago and back in Mexico. In the mid-1980s, street gangs were notorious, but their influence seems to have subsided in recent years, primarily as a result of community action.

In the 1980s Latino immigrants without documents tended to concentrate in the Near West Side. They go there looking for work in the small, locally owned factories and businesses. Although Mexican Americans have taken over the drywall trade in Chicago, jobs in this sector are not easy to come by and the attendant health risks, as yet unconfirmed, will probably prove to be high. The new arrivals from the southern border speak only Spanish and have few job skills other than those used in agriculture, but the will to work is strong. Many of these newcomers are initially homeless. It doesn't take them long to find El Centra Causa, a homeless shelter supervised by Sister Karen Bernhard of the Order of Humility of Mary. In 1988, Rush, which is only a few miles away from this shelter, created the Neighborhood Family Practice Clinic, with Dr. Steve Rothschild as medical director. At the start he had one full-time partner, Dr. Maria Brown. Because of the quality of care they provided, their reputation grew quickly, and in 1994 they were asked if they could provide some basic health care for those living in and using El Centra Causa.

Since RCSIP was emerging as an effective community service program, Dr. Rothschild invited me to a number of meetings with community leaders.

These meetings were eye-openers. Pilsen was going through a major transition. "Outsiders" were beginning to visit more frequently and in larger numbers. Pilsen had gained the identity of an "ethnic neighborhood" where Chicagoans and tourists alike could come for authentic Mexican cuisine, listen to the music of the barrio, and buy Mexican art and artifacts. Local business people, many of whom had been in the neighborhood all their lives, were beginning to worry that having El Centra Causa on the "main drag" was already a deterrent to visitors; now there would be a clinic that would attract even more homeless people. These were legitimate concerns that had to be worked out. It was a great exercise in community development through open discussion, negotiation, and compromise. What stood out was that all the stakeholders' positions were considered in reaching the final solution. It was agreed that some form of health care was needed for the homeless population in Pilsen.

Dr. Maria Brown, who speaks fluent Spanish, ran the clinic on Tuesday nights. She received backup from the Family Medicine Department at Rush. Once things were running smoothly, she began taking students for a series of rotations. Sister Karen supervised the operation and made sure the residents knew about the clinic and the opportunity to get free health care. To facilitate the project, Sister Karen conducted her own survey to determine the patients' major complaints—lots of infections, especially respiratory, as well as diabetes and what many thought were the symptoms of high blood pressure. She was aware that many suffered from alcohol and drug addiction. Besides beds and a good meal, El Centra Causa offered showers and a place to clean up. Clean clothing was distributed on a regular basis. The Pilsen Homeless Clinic, as it was known, was not located in the dormitory area; it was meant to be seen as a separate entity. In this way, Dr. Brown and her team were seen as offering a medical service that was independent of the shelter.

As the Pilsen Homeless Clinic evolved, a team of student volunteers, under Dr. Brown's watchful eye, provided basic primary care to the residents. Because there were only two small rooms that could be used for seeing patients, only a few students at a time could be accommodated in the clinic setting, and so Dr. Brown's approach was different from that at St. Basil's. All the students present participated in the diagnosis and treatment. Dr. Brown, the consummate teacher, got them involved according to their level of training. Third- and fourth-year students, who had more medical treatment experience, were to make the diagnosis and decide on the treatment plan. In this process, they served as teacher to the preclinical participants, whose opinions were also solicited and who were involved in some patient care. It was a marvelous interaction in which everyone taught everyone else. No one was looking over anyone's shoulder or

evaluating anyone in a typical assessment (grading) posture. The freedom of
expression that was afforded made the students feel comfortable and open. In
other words, they weren't afraid of being pimped in the classic clinical rotation
sense. Maria was the mother hen guiding them, questioning them, directing
them, so that when they finished at the end of the evening, the students had
learned a lot and felt that they had done something worthwhile. Since almost
none of the shelter's inhabitants spoke English, the clinic also provided the students a chance to sharpen their Spanish. Along with looking after patients' feet
(bunions, ingrown toenails) and controlling their high blood pressure and diabetes, the health care team offered counseling and practical advice. These are
people at the bottom of the social scale, and their plight touched many of the
students deeply.

Dr. Brown was a wonderful example for them. Her no-nonsense treatment,
her kindness and concern, her "informal seminars" about the struggles of the
homeless were quickly absorbed by the students. During the bitterly cold
Chicago winters, she continues to make trips to lower Wacker Drive, an underground street where homeless people huddle together for warmth and security,
to rescue any who accept her help. The experiences for those students who
accompany her paint a vivid picture of what it is like to be down and out in a
major city.

Rob McKersie, now a family physician, became attached to the clinic and
continued to volunteer during his residency. Rob, like Peter, was older, in his
early thirties, when he matriculated at Rush. He came with a long history of
voluntary community service that included initiating, directing, and overseeing a theater workshop for young women incarcerated at the Cook County Jail
for Juvenile Offenders. He is married, has two young children, and practiced
family medicine in a South Side public health clinic until recently. He now
practices in Lawrence, Massachusetts. Here is his reflection on volunteering in
Pilsen under Dr. Brown's tutelage:

> I was very active in RCSIP. I chose one site, the homeless shelter in
> Pilsen, and stayed active at this site during my time at Rush. I volun-
> teered one half day a week while in medical school and would occa-
> sionally drop in during my family practice residency training.
>
> I chose the homeless shelter in Pilsen for two reasons. The first was
> that it allowed me to work with Dr. Maria Brown, who I feel is one of the
> best and most compassionate physicians I have met. Second, more than
> any other RCSIP program that I was aware of at any time, the homeless
> shelter in Pilsen allowed the volunteers (medical students and residents)

to assume significant responsibility in the patient's care. Right from the get-go, Dr. Brown—under her watchful eye—allowed us to examine, diagnose, and treat the patients. We were medical students who were forced to think and act like residents, and the residents were forced to think and act like attendings. The experience was invaluable to my training at Rush. No other experience until I was well into my third year furthered my understanding of clinical medicine and the art of healing more than the work I did at the homeless shelter in Pilsen.

Another valuable part of RCSIP is the obvious—it fulfills the need of medicine to have people serve the underserved. In a country where one in five people has no health insurance—and little access to health care— RCSIP is helping to offer care and compassion to the uninsured at no cost. RCSIP, in a small but important way, is helping alleviate the health care woes of this country.

In addition, RCSIP offers volunteers who were committed a chance to be around like-minded people—whose goal is to make medicine more accessible to all. Having a chance each week to interact with students, residents, and attendings that were of the same social philosophy was very engaging and invigorating.

Finally, I am of the opinion that what is learned early is carried on. Having programs like RCSIP available to medical students teaches them, at the earliest and most impressionable years of their medical training, the importance of volunteering and "giving back" to the community. I am a firm believer that this behavior, if learned early, is carried on in later years of one's profession.

In 1997 the clinic moved to a new facility, a church-sponsored community center with social services on Seventeenth Street. By this time the shame engendered by the term *homelessness* had subsided and the clinic began serving mothers, children, and families who were in dire straits, that is, the new homeless. The clinic has clearly demonstrated that, by serving the homeless and disenfranchised, it plays an important role in maintaining the well-being of the least fortunate members of the Pilsen community.

Besides the physical problems of the homeless, the students saw the social and psychological problems. A Rush professor of psychiatry, Dr. Stephanie Cavanaugh, provided psychiatric consultation, which was received quite favorably by the community. Without leaving Chicago, the students were having a "third world" experience. They felt the discomfort of being outsiders in their own hometown. Even though their patients could be categorized as "Mexican

Americans," they were not yet acculturated Americans, and they had a very difficult time adjusting to the weather, job opportunities, and the Americanization
of the Mexican culture that constituted their national identity. The students
were astounded by the gap between the new arrivals and the old-timers.
Although there was dissatisfaction from those at the top of the social hierarchy,
the community eventually accepted *los hermanos* from their native land. Over
time, these new arrivals, mostly men but some women and children also,
became more assimilated to the community. Currently, RCSIP's presence in
Pilsen is well known and respected.

The Franciscan House of Mary and Joseph

With the exception of St. Basil's, the clinics where RCSIP volunteers worked
are located within a three-mile radius of Rush. This was by design, not chance.
I took the students who had approached me about continuing some form of
community service at the end of my course in 1988 to the top of the hospital
parking garage so they could look out over the vast Near West Side. As part of a
study on the prevalence of high blood pressure in the inner city in the early
1970s, I had conducted a census of the Mile Square neighborhood, which is just
on the other side of the Eisenhower Expressway and within walking distance of
Rush. Like many large urban medical complexes, Rush and its companion
institutions are surrounded by areas that are home to poor people of color who
have little or no access to the modern medical service system, with the exception of the county hospital. This irony weighed heavily on the students' conscience. In our many talks, it was widely agreed that this should be our primary
area of concentration.

If you drive west down Harrison Street for about ten minutes past the
Illinois Medical District, which consists of 560 acres, four academic medical
centers, six hospitals, twenty-two hundred hospital beds, a broad range of government agencies, and a technology park, you will find the Franciscan House of
Mary and Joseph, an emergency overnight shelter with 250 beds, 225 for men
and 25 for women.[5] Its mission reflects the spirit of Saint Francis of Assisi, to
"provide for basic human needs such as food, shelter, encouragement and assistance in creating a better life for the homeless and marginalized, especially
those who are underserved." The shelter is filled to capacity most nights, especially in winter. Each morning, after a hot breakfast, the residents are asked to
leave. The establishment of the Rush clinic at "the Franciscan," as the students
refer to it, deserves special attention. As RCSIP began to expand, I encouraged
those students who approached me looking for a site to seek out on their own
new places where they could offer service. But I also made it clear that this had

to be done in a careful and systematic manner with particular emphasis on a well-conceived plan, sensitivity to the group being approached, and an apparent indication of acceptance based on the service to be provided.

Beginning in his first year, Craig Garfield was dedicated to finding a way of helping the homeless. He contacted homeless shelters, neighborhood clinics, the Chicago Health Department, and a number of leads that developed from a kind of loose network of possibilities. He was relentless in his pursuit, but it was not easy. Prior to finding the Franciscan, he had to deal with a number of setbacks and dead ends. He was surprised by the number of homeless shelters that turned him down. The message was the same: setting up a clinic would complicate the normal routine of the shelter, where visitors get a hot meal, spend the night, and leave the next morning. The Health Department had its own procedures for helping the homeless, mainly trying to get them to use existing public health clinics or going to shelters periodically to check for TB, AIDS, or other communicable diseases. Academic health centers, such as Rush, wanted nothing to do with the homeless, and the unwritten rule was that if they showed up at the emergency room they should be sent to the county hospital across the street.

Craig's pursuit proved quite an education. He was misled, stonewalled by both public and private agencies, and in one case actually lied to about a potential site. But despite all the frustrations and obstacles, he remained committed to his goal of starting a free clinic at a homeless shelter. His perseverance paid off during his M2 year when he learned from Dr. Cynthia Waickus, a member of the Department of Family Medicine at Rush, about Anthony Dekker, a physician who worked independently in supplying medical services at the Franciscan homeless shelter. Dr. Dekker invited Craig to join him. Following his initial encounter, Craig knew that this was the place. He had no problem volunteering, because the need was so great. He brought along not only other medical students, but also some nursing students who were interested in the plight of the homeless as well.

When Dr. Dekker left the city for another position, Craig asked Dr. Waickus to become the physician advisor. Later Dr. Paul Hanashiro, a senior physician in emergency medicine, joined them. These two committed people served as the main physicians for the clinic. Through Craig's vigilance, the Franciscan became a new RCSIP program with many students lining up to participate.

Craig was a quiet and unobtrusive activist. Without fanfare, he did what he felt he had to do. Although I wasn't aware of how he was doing academically, I must admit I was surprised when I found out he was going to Harvard for his residency in pediatrics. After residency, Craig and his fiancée (who attended medical school at Harvard) came to Chicago, where he completed a Robert Wood Johnson Clinical Scholar Fellowship at the University of Chicago. They are married now and have two children. Craig had this to say about his RCSIP experiences and his career choice:

> I was pretty active [in RCSIP]. I spent some time at St. Basil's and, I think, doing a couple of "One Shot Deals" [the students' name for their school inoculation program] and then I really got swept up in the idea that we medical students had a lot of energy that, if focused, could make a differ-ence. It struck me during the white coat ceremony when I looked at all those students committed to caring for people and I thought if we had a positive outlet to funnel this energy through it would be phenomenal. I think at that time St. Basil's had a long waiting list and otherwise moti-vated people were being turned away or volunteering less than they wanted, so I naively thought there must be a better way.
>
> I started and participated in the Franciscan clinic. It is hard to articu-late in words [what RCSIP meant to me] with such distance from the actual time. I do not think it is an overstatement to say I would not have made it through medical school without RCSIP. RCSIP is one of the pri-mary reasons I chose Rush over . . . other medical schools I was accepted to. It gave me a place and community of like-minded people from which to gather support during medical school. It gave me perspective on the role of the physician in society and my future role in the profession. It helped me develop skills I already had or had in smaller amounts—orga-nizational skills, advocacy skills. And, of course, it introduced me to two fabulous human beings—Claudia and Ed, and with their support I was able to make it through those four years despite nearly failing courses, having terrible rotations, and being bogged down by feelings of inadequacy.
>
> I am not sure that I was influenced as much as I was supported. I came to medical school wanting to contribute to our society in a larger way, and I thought this profession would allow me to do it. RCSIP gave me a vehicle to do this with some legitimacy. I did realize while doing my work at the Franciscan that adult medicine was too far along the tra-jectory of human experience (and misery in this case) to make much of a difference so I focused on pediatrics as a career to try to get closer to the source and provide more preventive care. But I always knew my "call to service" was to care for people in our society on the margin. It had more to do with social justice, ideas of socialism, and the right of people to

live healthy lives as much as possible that made me want to go to medical school and be involved in RCSIP.

My clinical work today is still with uninsured children—I like caring for these children and their families. Just as each Tuesday night after working in the Franciscan, we rallied together and talked about the importance of connecting on a human level with people you might not ordinarily connect with, so too now I recognize how working with families and children who may not often have someone take an interest in their well-being and development is a very important thing for the child's growth and my own development as a physician and a human being.

What is especially meaningful from my perspective is how the spirit of Franciscan House touched the students and physicians who volunteered there. Their clinic was essentially in a hallway, and so medications, bandages, gauze, and the like had to be portable; the Rush team members brought a kit with them each time they went to offer their services. The patients would line up and come into the "clinic" one at a time. Some were follow-up visits for chronic diseases such as hypertension and diabetes. At the start only men came, but when the clinic was going for a while and seen as a real asset, women began to come as well.

The last time I contacted Craig when he was still a student, he had this to say about what his experience at the Franciscan meant to him and his fellow students:

> No one really cares about the homeless anymore. In fact, people not only have become immune to them—they despise them! They see them as crazies, druggies, terrorizors, nuts. A lot of this is true in one sense. But they are human beings in need. You would have to be an idiot to believe that simply providing limited medical care is an answer to their problems. But, for example, when I was there last Tuesday night, and after we had worked up all of the patients (lots of respiratory problems and TB; the shelter staff has tested positive) you have to walk through this big open bay with all of these men sleeping on cots and snoring blissfully. And you know that they are just like you and me; they are living, breathing human beings. No more, no less, and they deserve to be treated as such.

Craig, like many of the narrators in this book, defines the attributes that constitute humanism in medicine. Of particular significance was his passion for self-fulfillment through service as a dedicated and compassionate physician. He points out emphatically that he picked Rush over other schools where he was accepted because of RCSIP. Furthermore, by being with "like-minded people," he experienced a reaffirmation of his own personal values regarding the practice of medicine. His other skills, administrative and interpersonal, were honed in the responsibility he accepted for starting a clinic at the Franciscan shelter. For Craig, the care of children was the right conduit for practicing medicine, since it gave him a channel for patient education and disease prevention. Serving poor and uninsured families enabled him, in his own words, "to connect on a human level with people you might not ordinarily connect with."

CommunityHealth

CommunityHealth is a volunteer-based free clinic on the Near West Side located about two and a half miles north of the Illinois Medical District.[6] The first site was on Ashland Avenue, close to Rush. Its founder and promoter, Serafino Garella, MD, called it a really dark and uninviting place, but when he started CommunityHealth in 1993 there was no money, just goodwill and commitment from him and his fellow physicians at St. Joseph's Hospital. Dr. Garella, besides being a fine clinician, was the head of the Department of Internal Medicine at St. Joseph's and a popular teacher. RCSIP students were the first to contact him about participating in this new free clinic, and he welcomed them with open arms. At present, CommunityHealth is in its third location, at 2611 West Chicago Avenue, and is open every day except Sunday and three evenings a week. The clinic brochure proudly announces its statistics: more than 17,000 patient visits, almost 13,000 free prescriptions, a huge cast of medical students and residents, 350 other volunteers, and close to $850,000 worth of pro bono services.

The facility at CommunityHealth is so superior to St. Basil's that it was a shock to the Rush students and their physician mentors when they first arrived. In fact, the clinic, with its fully equipped examining rooms, well-stocked pharmacy, and modern laboratory for in-house analyses, was better than many of the public health clinics the students had visited during the community health course. CommunityHealth serves as a model for free clinics in Chicago (and probably the country as well). When the students and I asked how such a magnificent clinic was possible, we learned that once CommunityHealth was making a name for itself as a major source of health care for the uninsured, Dr. Garella, on the basis of his reputation and public relations skills, was able to raise funds, especially from prominent individuals and corporate donors. In the process he was able to establish an organizational structure that included a professional fund-raiser.

The students were clearly impressed, but questions about community empowerment based on what they had learned from their other clinic experiences began to surface. From my own conjecture about this situation, I concluded that for the local community, because of its fluidity—new immigrants arriving on an almost daily—it was a godsend, since so many patients didn't speak English and CommunityHealth was their only access to quality primary care. It was accepted knowledge that CommunityHealth was the primary source of care for a number of undocumented immigrants who had come up from Mexico or Central America seeking work in Chicago and had eventually settled in a newly emerging Spanish-speaking community that was spreading north from the Medical District. The students were also exposed to a different ethnic and cultural population from those in Pilsen, a large new younger generation of Latino origin who were recent arrivals. Furthermore, the students became aware of an elaborate network of gatekeepers, extended families, and neighborliness that made the new immigrants feel welcome. The students witnessed a process in which a community was growing right before their eyes. They saw that finding jobs, pooling assets, and sharing apartments and rooms and even beds were part of a communal belief in hope and perseverance. More significant, they were privy to the creation of a social structure and the community network necessary not only to survive but also to grow and expand.

Rush students were assigned a Wednesday evening primary care clinic. Student teams, supervised by Dr. Andy Zalski and a group of family physicians from Illinois Masonic Hospital, at that time home of the Rush family practice residency training program, served as primary health care providers. Dr. Zalski and his colleagues used the triage and diagnosis/treatment that had been effective as a model developed at St. Basil's. What distinguished Rush students from those of other medical schools who came later was the voluntary basis of their commitment. An additional benefit, like that at Pilsen, was their being able to practice their Spanish.

One student who was especially active stands out for each clinic. For CommunityHealth that person was Niraj Laksham Sehagal, an internist who did his residency at Stanford and later pursued a career in preventive medicine at the School of Public Health in Berkeley. His narrative touches on the broader issues that face medicine today:

[For my master's in public health] I was in a small interdisciplinary program comprised mostly of physicians who all had similar "social conscience" leading them back for further education. I gave a couple of presentations last year and one at an alum banquet at the end of the year discussing the dichotomy between "public health" and the "medical model" around disease prevention and health promotion. Sadly, there is not enough integration between the two (as you well know) and Berkeley is one of the few places in the country that has a joint MD/MPH program that is actually based in the school of public health (rather than the medical center). I can think of several faculty members there who would share your sentiments.

One of the things I realized during my MPH year is that there are similarly talented people who work in both public health and medicine and many of them don't appreciate what the other is bringing to the table. Most of the people who live in the ivory towers of medical centers don't even know the role of many public health folks, whereas many of the public health folks spend tremendous energy putting down all physicians as money-focused, ego-driven slime that represent the problem. Public health and medicine continue to be far too distant from one another. I've always felt that it is very difficult to put the necessary and appropriate "social and community slant" on medical education because in our country medical care is not a social good (as compared with many places like Europe). [Doctors] are trained to understand the financial aspects of health care delivery rather than realizing this important truth. We don't make people healthy and change their risky behaviors by getting them into a doctor's office. We get them healthy by going into their communities and into their homes, giving them clean water, a job, safety, etc.

If you are socially minded (and trained to think that way!), you no longer simply treat your diabetic patients with medications without understanding all of the other issues in their lives, and home, and culture. Our leader[s] in DC [don't] have a clue.

I participated in RCSIP through all four years of medical school with greater voluntary commitment and leadership roles over time. Initially, I worked in two of the existing free clinics and also participated in other well-developed activities such as the HIV-education magic show. By my second year, I teamed with a few other students to help launch services at a third community-based health clinic. I was chair of the students' clinical steering committee and a member of the RCSIP executive committee. I received the James A. Schoenberger Award at graduation for outstanding achievement in health promotion and disease prevention from the Department of Preventive Medicine.

It is hard to give the "one" most valuable aspect of the opportunity to be involved in RCSIP. I think the ability of the program to remind you why you were needed as a physician and the importance of "health" promotion outside of a traditional doctor's office was certainly reinforced. It also gave immediate motivation to an otherwise gross amount of medical information in the first two years of school that has no context. Finally, it gave a broader sense of health and all of the players involved to make a system work. It also pushed you to think "outside the box" with traditional medical models of *disease* rather than *health*.

I think the RCSIP experience reinforced a social conscience I came into medical school with that I didn't feel was being utilized in the traditional educational format. It gave me a better appreciation of how to impact populations rather than individuals, health rather than disease and prevention rather than diagnosis.

In terms of career, I always wanted to be a generalist at heart. I think the medical educational system, particularly in academic centers, requires you to focus interests in a narrow fashion. This is often the challenge I face trying to do the best for the most people but knowing I still have to generate a salary through patient care or specific grant funding. My goal is to demonstrate how to incorporate public health principles in the practice of hospital-based quality care.

Niraj is certainly an academic physician at heart. It is interesting to see that he wasn't satisfied with the conventional medical-model approach to health care. RCSIP reinforced his social-over-individual and health-over-disease perspectives. These programs were extremely important to him on a number of levels. Emotionally they gave him a sense of purpose. He evolved from the process, emerging as a person whom other students looked up to. His leadership qualities carried over to his graduate medical training. What is so exciting is that he wants it all—excellence as a practicing physician and the insights of a public health researcher. It is a true dialectic. Especially compelling is the fact that he brings his sensitivity to social conditions into the academic health center. He is the personification of what we hoped to accomplish in the health of the public (Showstack, Fein, and Ford 1992)—a research clinician with a social medicine orientation.

Niraj also represents a fundamental attribute of what RCSIP is all about. Like so many students, Niraj found that his role at CommunityHealth was a catalyst for him; that is, his biomedical knowledge, his dedication to doctoring, and his sense of social responsibility came together. Medicine was more than skills and techniques, it was a passion. This is why the values issue is so important if medicine is to remain a profession.

RCSIP participants "suffered" some from their success at CommunityHealth because it soon attracted medical students and faculty mentors from four other Chicago medical schools, and this meant that the particular presence of the Rush students was not given the recognition they had become used to. The situation provided an important issue to confront. Weren't we willing to share the glory? What made us more special than any other students or doctors? On reflection, these concerns were more of my making, and the newcomers really didn't bother the Rush students, who did feel, however, that a great opportunity had been missed when they weren't able to work more closely with students from the other medical schools.

An interesting anecdote sheds some light on this particular concern. A Rush faculty mentor told me the following story: Rush students and faculty share the general medicine clinic with participants from another Chicago medical school one night a week. Students from the other school are given academic credit for their participation and, therefore, are evaluated by their faculty preceptors. The Rush physician volunteer told me that when you walk into the clinic you see about three-fourths of the patients sitting on the Rush side. Moreover, when it gets to be around 9:00 P.M., those from the other school begin checking their watches because it's time to get ready to leave. The Rush team members, however, continue until they see the last patient, and that can be well after ten o'clock. Although he knows he is biased, my colleague says the Rush students and faculty exude enthusiasm and excitement. "Ed," he said, "they really seem to be having fun!"

The Role of the Clinical Preceptors

For RCSIP to deliver community-based health required student-faculty collaboration. From the start it was not a hierarchical relationship; that is, the physicians didn't supervise the students in the traditional medical education system of power and position. Instead, it was collegial and reciprocal. The faculty served as mentors to the students. The faculty members enjoyed working with the medical students within the structure of a free clinic because there was no administrative pressure on being productive by seeing as many patients as possible in a limited time frame. There are critics who say this is taking advantage of patients. That may be why the board member at St. Basil's got support for his attack on our motives. I believe in Richard Horton's (2007) assertion: "Good doctoring is about listening and observing, establishing a trusting environment for the patient, displaying authentic empathy, and using one's skills and knowledge to deliver superb care" (19).

The RCSIP clinic settings allowed the faculty to teach in a Socratic manner; the students were not afraid to ask "dumb questions" or offer honest opinions.

Students continually told me there was very little competition in any of the RCSIP clinic projects. The time and effort put in by the primary care doctors had its own payoff for their specialties in terms of a dramatic increase in the number of graduates seeking primary care residencies. The students had learned, firsthand, that primary care can be a fulfilling and rewarding career.

A teaching session led by a volunteer physician offers a good example. The patient, besides being diagnosed for a number of physical ailments, said she heard voices that told her not to trust anyone or let a man touch her (she was worked up by a female medical student), and she also made a clicking noise with her tongue. This patient was obese and unkempt as well and had strong body odor. The physician, Dr. Andrew Davis, an internist, asked the students if they had anyone in their extended families who was peculiar in any way. When they all acknowledged they did, he used this as an example that so-called weird people are not particularly uncommon. He further pointed out that the practice of medicine entails more than physical signs and symptoms and that emotional and mental behavior mattered as well. Dr. Davis's lesson dealt with the "total patient"—mind, body, and spirit. He explained that such an approach was not easy and required empathy and sensitivity, qualities essential to a physician. The students' undivided attention demonstrated the importance of this lesson as a vital part of their future practice style.

To get some other personal perspectives on what participation in RCSIP meant to students, I asked the two family doctors who had been volunteering since the beginning for their comments. As mentioned above, Dr. Maria Brown has overseen the clinic at the Pilsen Homeless Shelter since it was first established. Here are her comments about what participating in RCSIP means to her:

> From a very practical point of view, [I believe that] anyone who is afforded a medical education in this country owes a huge debt back to the society who nurtured them. Even if one just looked at matching funds from the public sector to medical college, let alone the less concrete gifts—we owe big-time. Since I am unlikely to find the cure for AIDS or create national policy, direct service is my venue.
>
> But why mentor students? It is slow, so why not just see patients? Because I am impressed with the inherent desire of the Rush students to heal and comfort, regardless of the person's ability to pay—based purely on the need. We can help people who are sick and hurting. So, we "just do it"—to borrow from Nike. Because the world doesn't need one more seminar, treatise, or research project documenting how hideously poverty intensifies poor health. (Either we are very stupid, or we should

have it down by now.) Because the students need to know that they are right in their instinct to help—all human forms bleed and weep the same, regardless of ability to pay or who they know. Because, when the students are not required to be there, and they know that they are not being graded, they become real. They ask genuine questions, and I can challenge their intellect without their being threatened—true discourse and learning burst out all over. Sadly, in our hypercompetitive, ego-driven world, this is not always the case elsewhere.

But here is the real deal. I long ago eschewed doing anything I don't enjoy. (Please don't tell my bosses.) I find the practice of medicine, boiled down to the basics of the interaction between the people involved, unencumbered by fears about HMO denials, a wonderful human interaction. We all walk away a bit more human when it is done right. Health has no price—it is valuable beyond measure. The RCSIP experience affirms that for students, preceptors, and patients alike.

So, in a nutshell—I, like most people, do what I enjoy. It's pretty simple, really. Thanks for asking me—I am honored that the students would mention me.

You can see why Dr. Brown is so loved by the students. She is real in every sense—what you see is what you get. And what you get is a competent, committed, unassuming doctor who gets great satisfaction from serving the homeless and disenfranchised. What makes her exceptional is that she practices ambulatory care outside the aegis of the academic medical center and brings students with her to share in the experience. The policy for ambulatory care in the majority of academic medical centers is to operate as an extension for delivering patients for specialized or technological procedures.

I have also mentioned Dr. Steven Rothschild earlier. He is the head of the section of community medicine in the Department of Preventive Medicine and associate professor in family medicine, and he had a lot to say about his experiences in RCSIP:

I became a RCSIP preceptor from its very inception. When the students came to us and described what they were proposing, you couldn't keep me from getting involved. This type of volunteer effort, getting them out of the medical center setting and into the communities where people live (and struggle to survive) is something I believe in passionately. I had already been involved with teaching community-oriented primary care to students as an M2 elective course. This was an opportunity to have the students put it into action.

[When it comes to how these experiences affected me], at the time, they didn't have that much impact on me. I would have said that I was still pretty idealistic and a passionate advocate for the medically underserved, and this was just a part of who I was. Plus I was already taking care of poor people every day, even without RCSIP.

Looking back, however, it is clear that the students helped preserve my idealism and passion. If so many of them hadn't continued to volunteer, year after year, and to start new programs, and to spend hours at the end of the day helping others . . . if I hadn't worked so closely with them . . . perhaps I would have lost much of my commitment. Let's face it: cynicism, burnout, reaction are all pretty common responses to the uphill struggle of trying to change the world for the better. These students won't let you get bitter, however—because they keep challenging you, keep asking questions, keep trying to make a difference. And you know, as a faculty member, you always try to stay at least a couple steps ahead of them! So RCSIP forced me to stay true to my personal mission as a physician, at least the one I set for myself twenty-five years ago: to be someone who served those who were least served in society and to make a difference in the lives of the most vulnerable. (Just reading the last sentence indicates just how much volunteering in RCSIP has meant to me personally.)

To be honest, I don't know what effect RCSIP has on the students [in the long run]. But here is my best guess: I would divide the students into three groups. Some were just passing through, just to get extra clinical experience, pad their résumés, and the like, and weren't all that committed to the social mission of the program. This was probably the smallest of the three groups, maybe 20 to 25 percent.

The second group is the most frustrating. They came into medical school idealistic, and they volunteered for RCSIP for the right reasons. And yet at the end of medical school, they entered the high-salary technical fields, with little evident passion or commitment and no signs that they would make volunteerism a lifelong habit. I keep hoping that I am totally wrong about this group and that down the road, after residency, maybe after the kids have grown, that these guys come back to the poor and medically underserved in their community and begin to look for ways to help. My perception is that this group makes up another 25 to 30 percent.

Fortunately, I believe that for at least half of the participants [the third group], RCSIP locks them into a model of being a physician that is grounded in altruism and our highest values. That's a pretty good rate, if you ask me.

I hate to put it in these terms, but here goes: I think we are in a fight for the souls of these young men and women. Unless we offer them a way that they can make a difference in the lives of people that the health care system ignores or writes off . . . unless we show them how even a homeless guy lying on a mattress on the floor of an old warehouse is a guy with a family, and hopes and aspirations, and people he loves . . . unless we have these opportunities for students, the vast majority of them will graduate to become technically skilled, well-compensated, nice people who will never make a real difference in their communities. RCSIP helps preserve that idealism and energy and creativity that brings students to medical school in the first place.

It is clear that Dr. Rothschild has given considerable thought to what RCSIP represents, not only for the patients, clients, and students, but also for himself. The moral and ethical struggle within medicine troubles him deeply—his entire life has been devoted to social justice in health care. His middle group—the idealists who succumb to medicine as a series of specialty procedures—worries him the most. They worry me as well. They are pulled so powerfully away from those values that initially inspired them to want to be doctors that it is almost impossible to overcome the magnetism. In addition, they want the "good life," as promoted by a culture that is based on material and market principles. Most of them don't want anything ostentatious, just a good car, a nice home, vacation time, and a family. And why not? According to the norms of our postmodern culture, they acquired their success the hard way—they earned it. Moreover, they resent the idea of shrinking from their duties and responsibilities. *Duty* has become a dirty word; it is viewed as a form of conscription.

These two physicians—seasoned practitioners of community-oriented primary care—gave their honest appraisal not only of the students but of their experiences as well. They love guiding these idealistic young doctors-in-the-making, but the service side of the experience continues, after all these years, to have a strong effect on them. Serving the poor and uninsured is satisfying, worthwhile, meaningful, and ethical. The physicians who volunteer do so for the same reasons the students do; they see this simple act of caring as their obligation and responsibility. This continuity is the thread that keeps values central to medicine alive not merely as a mission statement of some institution or organization but as the very essence of proffering health care.

Although the St. Basil's partnership, as well as later ones at other clinics, were by definition ambulatory and primary care experiences, on occasion patients required further assessment or had to be hospitalized. At a private institution such as Rush, advanced diagnostic procedures and extended in-patient care had to be covered financially by insurance or in some other way. Many of the patients seen at St. Basil's did not even have Medicaid and there was no source of payment that they could rely on. We were aware that the underlying philosophy of St. Basil's was unrestricted free care.

Three residents from internal medicine who began volunteering at St. Basil's called an emergency meeting with the RCSIP leaders. They explained that not being able to hospitalize a patient at Rush was not only a terrible dis-advantage but a violation of their duty to "do no harm." After personal reflec-tion and serious discussions they felt that the only appropriate thing for them to do was disengage from their clinic participation. When they finished their presentation, a long and impenetrable hush fell over the room. When the resi-dents left, one senior student remarked, "They just don't understand urban medicine." What he meant was that the RCSIP participants knew they could not easily admit patients to Rush or other private institutions, so they used pub-lic health clinics for more advanced procedures and Stroger (Cook County) Hospital for hospitalizations.

Although they were dedicated in their commitment, the internal medicine residents had a very narrow view of hospitalizing a patient. They saw it only from the receiving side and had no notion of how to negotiate the admission process. In this regard, the students were one up on them. Regardless of this one incident, which was basically an administrative hang-up, I can't overem-phasize the rapport between the physicians and the students. There was a def-inite synergy in the teacher-student collaboration. It broadened their collective experience with the underserved, it helped in humanizing the patients, it was instructive in understanding the medical system and obstacles to care, it built confidence.

I also have the reflection of Dr. Erich Brueschke, the dean of the medical school during most of the period:

> First, as the chairman of family medicine and as a residency director for seventeen years, and then as dean for six years, I watched with delight the expanding community service, increased number of women and minorities at Rush Medical College, and the greater number of students choosing general medicine during Ed Eckenfels's and Claudia Baier's tenure.
>
> When students enter medical school, virtually all are focused on doing good, making a contribution to humankind, and living a meaning-ful life. They are then faced with an educational system that focuses on

knowledge, measurable objectives, and performance skills. The really important influences tend not to be measurable and are frequently too "soft" to make a difference to faculty. Leadership must promote an educational system that measures not only knowledge and abilities but also attitudes and provides valuable experiences as well.

Students are eager to learn to be the best physicians. When we emphasize only facts and procedures, we run the risk of dampening or even destroying those beliefs and attitudes that brought them to medicine in the first place. Faculty is enriched by exposure to fresh student attitudes.

What Ed and Claudia and a few others did was bring real patient influences to students, using student-run experiences that enhanced attitudes as well as created new appreciation for patients as individuals in a sea of the problems of life. The results of student-run clinics with broad but limited faculty support have made a great difference to our medical students and their abilities as future physicians. This approach can be readily replicated and has numerous merits.

RCSIP and the Four Clinics

When I look at the four clinics as a whole, with the wisdom of hindsight, I recognize certain congruencies that contribute to the fullness of RCSIP and its unique way of fostering idealism and virtue in the lives and careers of the student participants. First, with the exception of St. Basil's, the clinics were located in the immediate area surrounding the medical center. This was one of their goals, to serve those communities within the shadow of Rush and its companion institutions. Second, the patients who were seen ranged across a broad cultural and ethnic spectrum. At St. Basil's, it was working poor, unemployed welfare recipients, mostly African Americans from a decaying neighborhood. At the Franciscan, it was homeless men, some of whom were only passing through until they found work, and displaced women, many of them in their thirties and forties but looking as though they were fifty and over. At Pilsen, it was the homeless, including people who had been in the community for many years, as well as undocumented immigrants, mostly from Mexico, who were looking for a place to sleep and a meal until they too found work. At CommunityHealth it was mostly recent arrivals from Latin America, working hard to support their families but, in most cases, without health insurance. For all of them free care was a blessing.

Third, if you put the clinics on a continuum in terms of the quality of the facility, St. Basil's would be at one end, CommunityHealth at the other. What St. Basil's lacked in modern equipment and spaciousness it made up for in spirit. That's not to imply that CommunityHealth was less committed to providing free health care to those who needed it. All four clinics are founded on a belief in serving those who are left out of the existing system, whereby not only their health and well-being are addressed, but also they are seen as human beings and members of society. The two clinics for the homeless would be somewhere in the middle, best characterized by adding a health care service that in some small way could improve the lot of those who had fallen between society's cracks. Fourth, there are the values that underpin each clinic. St. Basil's seems almost absolutistic in its philosophy, as indicated by the name Free People's Clinic. Unfortunately, by holding RCSIP to this gold standard, some rigid board members misunderstood the good that was being done as a sign of self-aggrandizement. Franciscan House of Mary and Joseph, a homeless shelter based on the tenet of Christian charity, saw the RCSIP volunteers as full participants in that process. Pilsen Homeless Clinic was a direct response to community need. Dr. Maria Brown accepted the challenge of meeting that need. Trained at Cook County Hospital, fluent in Spanish (including some Mexican dialects), and enthusiastic and humbled about being a doctor, with no fanfare, she was there to give service. CommunityHealth, probably a model free clinic for the nation, saves the taxpayers millions by broadly meeting the health needs of an entire community.

I served on the board of St. Basil's Free People's Clinic; Claudia had a similar position on the board of CommunityHealth. The aim of both clinics was to serve the communities where they were located. In discussions with patients waiting to be seen in the general-medicine clinic at St. Basil's, they had nothing but praise for the RCSIP doctors and students who served them. During the three years in which the prenatal project was in operation, it was seen as an answer to a prayer. Regardless of how hard we tried to dissuade them, the young pregnant women referred to the Rush students as their doctors or, if pushed, their student doctors. Newborns were named after the students who provided the prenatal care. One wall in the clinic was filled with photos of the babies.

CommunityHealth was also a true community institution—started, maintained, and expanded by the people—with the help of concerned doctors and students. It was apparent that a good proportion of the clinic's clientele were illegal immigrants. (This was long before the current heated political debate.) Almost half the people who used the clinic on a regular basis spoke little or no English. But it was the warm welcome and sincere appreciation that made the students feel they were part of a fabric that constitutes a coherent community. This sense of belonging became a great source of satisfaction for them. The patients were especially responsive to the students who could relate to them in Spanish. As a member of the board of directors Claudia was able to confirm the students' belief that RCSIP was making a real contribution.

Both the Pilsen and Franciscan clinics were the only source of health care for the homeless who used these shelters. Without RCSIP doctors and students they would have been left to take care of their own health problems. An overlooked aspect of the provision of medical services was that it took pressure off the actual communities where the shelters were located. In other words, without the clinics as a source of intervention, very sick homeless people would be roaming the streets and alleys unattended.

Chapter 3

The New Faces of AIDS

**A virus was invading the culture. No one
knew why. You just prayed it didn't get you.
Tony Kushner's great drama "Angels in
America" has brought these memories flood-
ing back, and they break like waves on the
shores of a much-changed reality.**

—Dudley Clendinen, "AIDS after 'Angels': Not
  Gone, Not Forgotten"

In 1991 I attended a two-day symposium on AIDS at the New York Academy of
Medicine. I got an academic rate at a boutique hotel across the street from the
Metropolitan Museum of Art on Fifth Avenue. It was a beautiful late summer
day, so I decided to walk along Central Park to the academy. Everything was
still in bloom, the air was fresh and clear, the sun warm and comfortable; it was
one of those perfect days you wish could last forever, but at the same time you
know summer is almost gone. Bicyclers glided under the parkway bridges; kids
played soccer with a serious attitude; and the grassy knolls provided quietude
for people deeply involved in their reading, eyeing each other romantically, or
simply resting.

Once inside the academy I was assaulted by the reality of AIDS. One of the
first things that became apparent was the diversity of the audience. The pale
academics with their suits were obvious, but a large proportion of the capacity
crowd in attendance was different. There was a vast array of people of color,

mostly brown-skinned Latinos but a number of blacks as well. There was clearly a contingent of gays and lesbians who could easily be identified by their conversation and behavior. A few had the visible signs of AIDS—sunken cheeks and brown skin lesions. Young sexy Puerto Rican girls with tattoos, enormous earrings, and facial metal talked incessantly among themselves. This certainly wasn't a formal academic presentation—it was a happening!

The two days of sessions were amazing. It was not just what I learned (which was tremendous) but the feeling I got, the emotions I felt, the empathy and bonding that overwhelmed me. As Paul Farmer and Arthur Kleinman (1989) have said, "If we minimize the significance of AIDS as human tragedy, we dehumanize people with AIDS as well as those engaged in the public-health and clinical response to the epidemic. Ultimately we dehumanize us all" (139). What I saw made it impossible to minimize its significance.

There are two occurrences in particular that I want to mention from this experience. Two New York Public Health epidemiologists gave a brief but stark presentation about the transition from the "gay plague" to "dirty needles" and "straight sex." I viewed them as two New York Police Department narcotics detectives simply giving us "the facts, man." The story of the discovery of AIDS among intravenous (IV) drug users in 1983 was a real shocker. Monthly mortality and morbidity reports showed a tripling in the deaths of male vagrants, with the curve rising. Besides having needle marks on their bodies, almost all the men were emaciated, and since most were diagnosed as dying from pneumonia, it was assumed they might represent a potential epidemic of TB and related respiratory ailments. Because the increase was so dramatic, autopsies were eventually performed. These men had not died of ordinary pneumonia but, rather, a rare form, pneumocystic pneumonia, the result of the breakdown of the immune system. Another opportunistic infection was found, Kaposi's sarcoma, consisting of tumors of the skin that left brown splotches on the body and face. In short, this was full-blown AIDS. The epidemiologists had been invited to speak on New York's number-one talk radio station, WOR, to present their findings. The switchboard was bombarded with hundreds of callers. Most ranted with comments such as "Great, now we can finally get rid of those scumbags!" When it was discovered that the expanding epidemic included not only IV drug users, but also a wider population of women and straight males, the public who use the airwaves gave the same hostile response: good riddance.

The other incident was more personal and dramatic. A social worker showed a video of a session she had conducted with a young woman. She was talking to a beautiful Puerto Rican girl, no more than twenty years old, about living with her boyfriend, who was HIV seropositive. Gently but firmly she kept telling her (call her Maria) that she had to leave him or she, too, would become infected. There was fear, anger, and resolution in Maria's replies: "Man, you don't get it. . . . I know all about that AIDS shit, but I don't even know where the fuck I am going to sleep tonight. . . . Besides, man, I'm garbage, I'm rotten, and the only thing you do with garbage is bury it." This brought out lots of comments from the young women in the audience. They talked about safe sex, multicolored condoms, watching out for each other. They were a powerful force for prevention through education. It was amazing. Most of the women started their statements with "Hi, I'm Rosa. I have AIDS." Many of them talked about the Colombian drug lords living in the Mott Haven section of the Bronx who tried to pimp them all the time by offering fancy clothes, nights in luxury hotels, and the "good life." I had encountered a "new" social class—women with AIDS.

The gays and lesbians among those present had two themes: the increasing and vast majority of those dying from AIDS were gay and public awareness and any government response was the result of the strong stand they took through the actions of organizations such as ACT UP (AIDS Coalition to Unleash Power), a diverse, nonpartisan group of individuals united in anger and committed to direct action to address the AIDS crisis. On the national level, more than 107,000 cases had been diagnosed and more than 62,000 deaths (more than in Vietnam) had been recorded by 1988. Not until 1990 did former president Ronald Reagan actually use the terms *HIV* and *AIDS* publicly.

What touched me most deeply in this free-for-all were the human suffering and the willingness of people with AIDS and their lovers, families, and friends to discuss it openly. The New York experience was the first time the full impact of AIDS struck me. I admit it had been an abstraction, a series of vital statistics, and an "isn't that terrible" attitude. Within the next couple of years at least five people I knew, two personally, died of AIDS.

As I flew back to Chicago, I thought about the concern RCSIP members had already expressed regarding the need to develop some way of addressing AIDS. I couldn't help but admire the way the students had reacted spontaneously to this devastating crisis. In fact, we learned that some students not only knew someone with AIDS but also someone who had died from the affliction. Gay and lesbian students were afraid of saying anything because they feared it would reveal their sexual identity. There were no gay or lesbian organizations in medical schools at that time. Most homosexuals seeking a career in medicine remained closeted, especially when blood was found to be one of the major fluids of transmission.

In our initial discussions regarding the creation of RCSIP, we gave considerable thought to what medical students, most of whom were still in their preclinical phase of training, could actually do. It was decided that the best means of reaching the largest number of people was through disease prevention and health-promotion activities. Although these approaches have become a cliché as presented in textbooks and lectures on preventive medicine, this was not the case with the RCSIP designers. The students were quite aware of the limitations of what they could do in clinical settings. Nonetheless, prevention and health education could be performed outside the clinic, in settings such as schools. AIDS offered a significant opportunity in this regard. In retrospect, they were ahead of the curve.

RAIDS

By the start of the 1988 school year, the medical students knew that the AIDS epidemic had taken a new direction; it was no longer referred to as the "gay plague." The HIV virus was now being transmitted through the sharing of dirty needles among IV drug users and through the exchange of body fluids from an infected person to his or her sexual partner, including transmission between heterosexuals. AIDS patients were starting to be admitted to Rush. Attending physicians, residents, nurses, and the rest of the clinical staff were learning how to care for them. The infectious disease section was conducting clinical trials on new drugs. The basic scientists in the Department of Immunology were involved in laboratory research. AIDS was on everyone's mind and was now a topic in the curriculum. This new epidemic, however, was carefully crafted to fit into the biomedical paradigm.

But RCSIP wanted to play its own role in the new epidemic. The offshoot was RAIDS—Rush (students fighting) AIDS—which was in the planning stage two years before my trip to New York. Outside of abstinence, safe sex and clean needles were the only forms of prevention. The logical question that evolved was, How can AIDS prevention and safe sex be taught to sexually active high school kids? RAIDS planners started by outlining three components of inquiry: What did the high school kids need to know? What kinds of questions would they ask? and How could the presentations be made interesting? At about that time, I was contacted by the principal of a high school for adults; these students had dropped out of school, some as many as ten years before, and returned to get a "real" high school diploma rather than the general equivalency diploma (GED). The progressive-minded principal felt that they needed some health education for the "real world of sex" as well. In particular, she was interested in having someone talk to these young adults about AIDS. She was referred to us by a personal friend who knew that we wanted to get involved with the disease at some level.

Before any teaching actually took place, the RCSIP members began focusing on a curriculum. They created a course syllabus that was introduced at the American Medical Students Association and eventually served as a stimulus for the organization to develop a standardized outline that could be used at all medical schools. The students prepared themselves by going over topics; by practicing keeping presentations simple, interesting, and to the point; and by using anatomy models as visual aids during their talks. They got faculty from infectious disease to teach them how AIDS was transmitted. The students tried to anticipate every possible question. For example, can you get AIDS from a mosquito bite, from French kissing, from saliva, a toilet seat, and the usual suspects?

David Pate, from the Ounce of Prevention program and member of the Department of Preventive Medicine, spent a number of sessions teaching the medical students how to "talk the talk" about sex with inner-city kids and adolescents.[1] He pointed out that broaching the topic of sex was not easy for either party. The medical students would be challenged with a lot of four-letter words and inner-city jive. In my sessions, I used data from the Guttmacher Institute showing that unwanted pregnancies among teenagers had been lowered significantly in some Scandinavian countries when teachers, using models, actually showed students how to put on a condom and what was actually involved in other forms of safe sexual behavior. If they didn't have the appropriate models, they could improvise—put a condom on a banana.

Of course, being medical students, they devoured every bit of information, data, and procedure they were taught. They were highly successful in the special high school partly because the students were older and more mature (a few were older than the medical students). The women in particular were frightened of getting AIDS. One icebreaker of these early sessions was to ask if they knew of anyone who was HIV positive or had AIDS. The medical students were surprised at how many hands went up. (In a few years they would be asking the same question among themselves or if they knew anyone who had died from AIDS.) They also used games such as passing out envelopes to the students in which only one contained a "Yes" referring to having AIDS. Then they had them pass the envelopes around the room. When they stopped the rotation, they asked how many had received a Yes card. In less than ten minutes everyone had. The RCSIP teachers used this device to demonstrate the exponential spread of the disease.

The word must have got out through teacher networks because, on the basis of their success in this setting, RCSIP students were invited by concerned teachers and principals from public schools to conduct AIDS education and prevention programs in inner-city high schools where sexual activity was widespread. Getting started was the most difficult part. The medical students were anxious about running into a hostile attitude: who are these white dudes to come into our neighborhoods and lecture us? Initially, the medical students were hit with notions about sex that were outside their frame of reference: "After sex, a douche with a well-shaken Coke killed all the sperm, so wouldn't it kill the AIDS virus?" "Rubbers don't make for good sex." "If you look at the people dying of AIDS they are all fags." Black gay men were called "fairies" in their neighborhoods and were considered the opposite of the macho male. The female students were most receptive at first. They didn't want to get pregnant, let alone get AIDS.

Rapport developed more quickly than I expected. Two things seemed to hit home: what the virus did to you regardless of how healthy or strong you were and the mechanics of practicing safe sex. A lot of laughing and joking, by all parties, masked anxiety and fear. Through these informal, interactive, and open discussions, the RCSIP participants focused on ways of getting the classroom audience to understand how their sexual practices and the IV use of illicit drugs could affect their health, lives, and well-being. In addition, by focusing on prevention, the medical students stressed the human need to treat people afflicted with AIDS with sensitivity and understanding. Since they were medical students, I reminded them to keep the immunology and infectious disease part at a minimum and focus primarily on the human side of AIDS. Pre- and posttests were used as a rough estimate of their impact, and continuity was maintained through follow-up sessions. The overall ignorance about sex and the sexual transmission of disease, as well as disease outcomes, was overwhelming. Posttest answers and follow-up discussions indicated that the youngsters had become much better informed.

In the final analysis it was the medical students' enthusiasm and candor, based on Pate's training and their deep conviction about what they were doing, that enabled them to engage in open and free-flowing discussions with the high school and middle school kids. The fact that they were not authority figures but were young and trusting helped the medical students. Both groups of students learned to respect each other, and that respect made the real exchange of critical information possible.

Meeting youngsters who were sexually active at such an early age without any health care resources besides the school nurse, along with myths of how to prevent pregnancy, was completely new for the medical students. In the middle of one session, a teenage boy said that the word in the "hood" was that "Jew doctors had invented AIDS to wipe out blacks, since they were having so many babies." This attitude was prevalent among many black kids for a while and posed a real test for RAIDS participants. It precipitated a new strategy aimed at debunking other myths about AIDS, including that of the "monkey virus." Confronting myths with science was tough but highly rewarding.

In sum, the medical students encountered firsthand the way misinformation and poor communication reinforce prejudice. During the first year alone RCSIP made presentations at five different schools. At more than one school, RAIDS became a standard part of the health education curriculum. The program ended, as a result of its own success, in 1994. The example set by RCSIP encouraged the board of education to introduce a real sex education program into the public schools. By that time, RCSIP's AIDS prevention and safe sex presentations had been heard by more than two thousand school kids.

The Rush Pediatric AIDS Support Program

As the AIDS epidemic became more prevalent, a particularly tragic outcome was the phenomenon of children who were born HIV positive. The prognosis of developing full-blown AIDS was high, resulting in death within a few years. The medical students wanted to find some way of helping these kids, but they didn't know where to start. We were aware that almost all the cases were being treated at Children's Memorial Hospital, the leading pediatric institution in Chicago. When RCSIP students contacted the hospital, they were told they could apply to become volunteers but there was a long waiting list. The RCSIP proposal involved more than being volunteers; they wanted to become "siblings" to the children. What they had in mind was spending special periods of time with them—going to the zoo, walking in the park, visiting museums—in short, being their friends. The medical students felt stonewalled.

But an interesting coincidence occurred. My wife was on the board of the Frank Lloyd Wright Home and Studio, and John Thorpe, the chief architect for the organization, had renovated a large prewar bungalow, the Children's House, to serve as a home for HIV kids. We were invited by John to the dedication ceremony. Mingling among the crowd was Dr. Ram Yogev, chief of the AIDS unit of the Department of Infectious Diseases at Children's Memorial. I approached him with the RCSIP proposition. He was aghast at the idea. He announced that there was no way medical students were going to learn about AIDS on his patients. He went on about the sensitivity and fragility of the children and how he and his specially trained staff had carefully screened and picked the volunteers. I told him about RCSIP and our AIDS education programs. The medical students had one aim and one aim only, to help the kids by being their friend and buddy.

This gave Dr. Yogev pause. He brought up lots of arguments: they will want to go on rounds, they will ask clinical questions, they will tend to see the children in terms of their biomedical training. No, that's not it, I replied. Right now, they are teaching AIDS in the inner-city schools; they get the fundamental aspects of AIDS as a disease in their preclinical courses; and, on the wards, they actually see AIDS patients. They simply wanted to reach out to these children and their families with love and care. His counterargument was that this could quickly turn maudlin. I explained that it was actually an act of altruism— an ingredient too often missing in physicians—that would help keep their idealism alive. Yogev made a pact with me. First, the students had to go through a very careful screening by the volunteers, the staff, the AIDS specialists, and, of course, the doctor himself. Concern by anyone involved would mean the student was out. Second, it was a commitment for the rest of their medical school education—too much was at stake to let the kids down.

Initially the clinic staff at the hospital was extremely cautious about the role the medical students were proposing. It was not unusual at that time for a child with AIDS to die shortly after diagnosis; therefore, their caregivers were especially protective. The original five Rush students had to work very hard to convince the staff, and Dr. Yogev in particular, that they were capable of making a real contribution to the lives of the infected children. The process was intense. The medical students had to win approval from the professional staff (child life specialists and social workers) as well as the volunteers. It was a thorough screening. In addition, they had to keep proving that their primary reason for wanting to volunteer was to help the children and not simply to learn about the pathophysiology of the disease. After going through the screening (a full day or more), the next stage took place in play sessions, run primarily by the volunteers. The children who participated in these events lived at home, and the play sessions functioned as a kind of "day hospital" when the children came in for evaluation. Initially, the medical students would simply hang around and play, read, or talk with the children. After a few sessions it became evident that a particular child was starting to bond with one of the medical students.

This was the beginning of the process but not the end. Each medical student also had to be accepted by the parent who came to pick the child up at the hospital and, eventually, the whole family, including siblings. This meant going to the child's home and meeting everyone. The foundation of the relationship between the big sib and his or her kid required the medical students to show their affection for the child. Their sincerity soon won everyone over. In addition, they were sworn to strict confidentiality about who the children were, details of their families, where they lived, and the like. But it was common knowledge at that time that most of these children were born to women who were IV drug users or whose male partner was an AIDS carrier. In their reflection on their sibs and their families, the students told us they had to be sensitive to any other children in the household. A host of emotions in the family dynamic were frequently expressed, from envy to dislike and fear, as in so much else in human interaction. The experience was more than one on one; it involved everyone in the child's background.

But through their persistence, open-mindedness, and honesty—demonstrating that they really wanted to do this—a group of five students were able to develop a trusting relationship with the hospital's staff and the children's parents. The Rush Pediatric AIDS Big Sib program (the students' title) doubled the number of students involved by the second year. Because of the emotional demands on all parties, this project required an especially strong commitment on the part of the medical students. Although this effort was not clinical in a strict medical sense, it illustrates the medical students' capacity to meet one of the greatest requirements in the care of children with AIDS—giving the love, nurturing, and stability these children so desperately need (Tess et al. 1997). During the first five years of the program many of the children died before the medical students graduated.

To the question of why students were willing to become a big sib to a child who was HIV positive, Peter, who is now a pediatrician, without hesitation, gave the following reply: "I love kids. Rudy has AIDS; he is going to die. I want to remain human and loving when I have to deal with the death of a child. It may seem selfish, but I simply can't wait until I am a full-fledged doctor. I know I have much to gain from him. I only hope that I am giving something in return."

Some might consider Peter's attitude as "selfish altruism." But altruistic acts always include oneself in some way. As Coles has observed, "You learn and develop through giving."

The AIDS Prevention Magic Show

The AIDS Prevention Magic Show reveals what ingenuity medical students have and how they can use their special talents when given an opportunity to do so. In fact, this project would surely never have come about had RCSIP not existed, and what an amazing innovation it was!

Stuart Lustig was a very unassuming young man when he arrived at Rush, but he soon showed us how dynamic he really was. While a first-year medical student, he created and instituted the AIDS Prevention Magic Show: Avoiding the Tragic with Magic. The show took about thirty minutes and was presented by Cyrus the Virus (portrayed by Stuart), a sinister but entertaining character who used magic tricks to explain why sharing needles and choosing sexual partners based on appearance alone can result in contracting HIV and eventually AIDS. Cyrus also used magic to communicate ways in which AIDS is not transmitted, how to refuse sex, and how to use condoms correctly. His main concern was establishing an understanding of healthy sexual behavior.

Initially the show was geared toward youngsters ten to fifteen years old, but because it was so well received, Stuart performed it before even younger children, eight to twelve. I witnessed a live show for preteens at the Boys and Girls Club in the Henry Horner housing project. Cyrus performed his magic before more than one hundred children prior to starting his clinical rotations. Because the show was fully scripted, he was able to train another ten medical students to become Cyrus (or Iris, if she were female) to continue the magic show after he graduated. Cost of materials was a little more than one hundred dollars, and so there were no economic barriers. He sold a number of "magic kits" to raise money to keep the program going.

The show begins with a trick called "Silly Silks," in which Cyrus shows that sharing needles transmits HIV; he made a red handkerchief, representing blood, disappear from a syringe and appear between two white handkerchiefs tied together, representing two friends sharing needles. "Missing in Action" is a card trick consisting of pictures of five ethnically diverse youths. Four of the pictures show "AIDS" printed on the back and the fifth shows "HEALTHY." The audience learns by trial and error that they cannot guess who is healthy simply by looking at the faces on the cards. When the last card is flipped, it now also shows "AIDS," indicating the risk to people who guess their partners' health status based on appearance alone. In "Reading between the Lines," black-and-white pictures in a coloring book show ways in which AIDS cannot be transmitted. Flowers made of colored condoms are waved over the book and the pictures become colored. Another wave of the flowers and the pictures turn into the words "USE CONDOMS." To improve perceived self-efficacy at refusing sex, "Just Say No! No! No!" is rehearsed by repeating three statements to use when refusing sex, statements that are printed on a condom-shaped card. When placed in an envelope and later removed, the third card bears a different response—the only one possible when one is out of condoms—it says, "No, No, No." In "Condominimum," the last trick, Cyrus discusses how to buy, store, put on, take off, and dispose of a condom, during which he pulls a condom out from behind the ear of a volunteer and later penetrates but does not burst an inflated condom with a sixteen-inch needle.

The AIDS Prevention Magic Show was so successful that Stuart was besieged with calls from all over the country either to appear in person or to prepare a protocol for performing the tricks. To accommodate the requests,

Stuart actually videotaped a show before a live audience and made it available for distribution. In 1994, he received a Secretary of Health and Human Services Award for Innovation in Health Promotion and Disease Prevention.

It is most interesting to compare this creative and engaging approach with how sex education is being taught in today's public schools. Getting youngsters to understand human sexuality and all its manifestations takes imagination and even humor, elements that are certainly missing in the formality and moralizing that constitute what passes for sex education for our children and adolescents today. The significance of this project, a great investment of time and energy, on Stuart's career in medicine is found in his narrative. He has since finished his residency training in psychiatry at Stanford, which was followed by a fellowship in child psychiatry at Harvard. His own words relate the full meaning not only of his project but also of RCSIP for the students:

> My experience developing, performing, teaching, and writing about the AIDS Prevention Magic Show was as much a part of medical school for me as studying for exams, dissecting a cadaver, and getting comfortable with patients.
>
> During the winter of my fourth and final year of medical school, I wrote to Dean Brueschke in support of RCSIP programs: "RCSIP was also a young researcher's boot camp for me. Ed and Claudia became my mentors and also brought on board a statistician, Steve Daugherty, enabling me to greatly enhance the validity of my survey instrument used to measure the [magic] show's success."
>
> While I learned more than most medical students about the importance of evidence-based interventions and research methods, I also grew to understand the importance of mentors to my professional, moral, and spiritual development. Ed and Claudia were my first mentors, and they held my hand as I took my first steps forward into my new profession and began to understand the importance of lifelong learning and my potential contribution to medical knowledge. As a child psychiatrist, I am fully aware of the parental attributes I have ascribed to Claudia and Ed, who were affectionately dubbed Mom and Dad by other RCSIP participants. With Claudia's unchecked enthusiasm for my RCSIP pursuits, and with Ed's laborious and insightful corrections to my writing, my defenses as a self-assured and autonomous medical student gradually gave way to a more meaningful collaboration with others and trust in the knowledge and guidance that comes from a warm, productive mentoring relationship. Their mentorship has continued as the standard to which

I compare other mentors. Their gentle and enriching guidance has been difficult to replicate, and it has inspired me repeatedly to work collaboratively toward professional pursuits with investigators and clinicians more seasoned than I, always resulting in greater gain.

In the same letter to the dean, I wrote: "When sleep is occasionally scarce and morale low at times, these [free] clinics give students the chance to remember why they chose to be doctors." I also served as a volunteer for the Erie Health Center, in which students have the chance to interview elderly patients at home to provide needs assessments of daily living. With the frequency of house calls rapidly declining, these valuable visits remind students of the circumstances in which patients live and function.

As a child psychiatrist in practice for about two and a half years now, I reread these statements and said to myself, "Yes! RCSIP's mission got through to me!" Looking back, I suspect that my participation encouraged my chosen career path. Psychiatrists, in general, and child psychiatrists, in particular, must, more than any other type of physician, understand the totality of patients' experiences. We know that the thirty-minute or sixty-minute patient snapshot in our offices may bear little resemblance to the rest of a child's day or week. As a consultant to four school systems, I have the opportunity to see firsthand the circumstances in which these children live and function, and to make adjustments to their environment by empowering the staff who work with them for several hours each day. It was under Ed and Claudia's tutelage that I first developed the understanding that schools provide a crucial interface for services and their intended recipients; with their guidance, as a medical student, I performed the AIDS Prevention Magic Show at numerous schools in Chicago.

RCSIP also helped me to develop a sense of loyalty to those in our society who cannot pay for or sometimes even access the care they deserve. Working in St. Basil's clinic in Chicago's South Side, dubbed by Jim Croce as "the baddest part of town," sensitized me to the brutal realities of many of the patients I have served through a career in public psychiatry. St. Basil's was the first in a long line of institutions, such as Massachusetts Mental Health Center, Boston Medical Center, and Cambridge Hospital, that collectively involved me with hundreds of patients who struggle just to keep an appointment because of poverty, isolation, and disenfranchisement.

Much of my recent professional work has focused on some of the most vulnerable among us, namely, unaccompanied child refugees and children in immigration detention who have been viciously traumatized, estranged from caretakers, and thrust into the utter unfamiliarity of our country's language and cultural practices. My ongoing involvement with Physicians for Human Rights and burgeoning collaboration with another advocacy organization, Amnesty International, no doubt results from the community service values I developed in RCSIP.

Stuart's account of his RCSIP experience leading to and exemplified in his career provide a strong sense of the attitudes and values that were cultivated and reinforced. Here are some of the most obvious: When he became Cyrus the Virus and reached kids who were primarily poor and black, he bonded with them; this bonding resulted in his commitment to dedicate his professional life to helping children. His selection of child psychiatry demonstrates awareness that there is more to an illness, even a mental one, than the biological data. It is a form of holism, which, for Stuart, integrates all aspects of a child's life. Here again, the humanistic connection takes place. Cyrus the Virus was Stuart's alter ego, that is, his humanism in action that would eventually meld with his medical knowledge and skills side. This is evident in his career as a socially active physician.

It is also gratifying for us to be seen as mentors not only in an emotionally supportive role but as competent professionals who maintained rigorous standards in our teaching and research. Finally, I would be remiss if I didn't emphasize the social responsibility side of Stuart's professional development. His values are evident in his psychiatric practice and in all facets of his life, as demonstrated by his affiliation with humanitarian organizations.

The Face Is Human

What do these AIDS-directed activities tells us about RCSIP? The short answer is, A lot. Once again, it is their ingenuity and passion that come bursting through. The RCSIP students absorbed the tragedy and changing faces of AIDS in their own way: teaching prevention through safe sex, adopting children who were suffering from the ailment, and making learning about its potential devastation something that youngsters could deal with—through fun and games.

The diverse group of people actively dealing with AIDS whom I met in New York had a profound effect on me by reaffirming the attributes I could bring to the AIDS planning discussion. As medical students, the RCSIP participants "glommed on" to the strictly medical components of AIDS—its pathophysiology, its etiology, its epidemiology with special focus on infectious diseases. It wasn't that they were insensitive to the attendant pain, suffering, and death, but, rather, the clinical construct lacked the social and ethical context of this horrendous epidemic. I pushed, related, or quoted from writings that were not strictly biomedical. For example, I referred to Mart Crowley's *Boys in the Band*; Susan Sontag's *AIDS and Its Metaphors*; and an issue of *Daedelus* devoted to the psychological, cultural, and social aspects of AIDS. This was always the students' and my struggle, that is, not to succumb totally to what Good (1994) calls the "medical gaze." Regardless of how philosophical I got, they always remained pragmatic but not at the price of losing their humanism.

The AIDS projects offer another insight into the spirit of RCSIP. After the first health education project at the high school for dropouts, all the health education—safe sex, AIDS prevention, human anatomy, health, and hygiene—conducted in the public schools was by request and based on the reputation of RCSIP participants. The medical students were recognized as great teachers who were receptive and open to sharing information. The fact that RCSIP was constantly receiving requests from schools, shelters, and community groups speaks to their credibility.

Over the decade of the 1990s I witnessed a major change in attitude about using medical students as service workers. Conventional wisdom was that this stuff is nice in high school or college, but now it is time to learn how to be a real doctor. This attitude change happened because the students were able to demonstrate they could make a real contribution in meeting community needs. An indication of their commitment was their willingness to go into communities where more established agencies would not enter or address a public health problem, such as AIDS, which was provocative and emotion laden. In their minds, the students were not sacrificing their biomedical education; they were broadening their perspective in keeping with the core values of the profession.

As in all RCSIP enterprises, the significance of community acceptance can't be overstated. In the final analysis the AIDS projects became accepted because they were real. In all these endeavors—RAIDS, Big Sibs, Cyrus the Virus—the students' compassion, sensitivity, and knowledge reached not only those they served, but also themselves and their mentors.

Chapter 4

Community-Based Grassroots Programs

It is not enough to provide accessible, cost-
effective, quality health care; the population
for whom it is intended—the community—
must have faith in its quality, and must feel
that their health is the primary concern of
that provider, that there is no ulterior
motive involved and that the providers are
sensitive to and knowledgeable about their
lifestyle and culture.

—Medical student, in Bridging the Gap
   program, 1997

There are two RCSIP programs that are essentially grassroots in nature. One
began at Henry Horner Homes, a Chicago Housing Authority project on the
Near West Side, and the other at Casa Guatemala, in the Uptown community
area on the Far North Side.

In 1935 as a building block of the New Deal, President Franklin D. Roosevelt
and Congress created the Works Progress Administration, later called the Works
Project Administration (WPA), for the primary purpose of getting the unemployed victims of the Great Depression back to work. Besides building national
parks, bridges, and new highways and supporting major works of art, the WPA
constructed public housing for poor families. The Chicago Housing Authority
(CHA) was made possible by the WPA and the Federal Housing Act of 1937. Prior
to World War II, four low-rise projects (two- to four-story buildings) were constructed on the Near West and South Sides. The Ida B. Wells Homes, one of the
first built, was strictly for blacks. This was the outcome of a policy, the so-called
Neighborhood Composition Rule, that laid the foundation for de facto racial

segregation and governed these developments in future years. Gerald Suttles (1968) writes about this in his classic study, *The Social Order of the Slum*.

During World War II, CHA was redirected to create housing for workers in war industries. After the war, CHA provided several thousand units of temporary housing for veterans and their families. In the 1950s and 1960s the new trend in public housing was to construct high-rise apartment buildings reaching sixteen stories. Built in 1962, the Robert Taylor Homes, the largest housing project in the United States at that time, consisting of 4,415 units in twenty-eight identical sixteen-story buildings, was spread from Thirty-ninth to Fifty-fourth Street along the Dan Ryan Expressway. By the late 1980s CHA was the third-largest housing authority in the nation, with more than 130,000 residents in approximately 67,000 units. If it were a city, in its heyday it would have been the second largest in Illinois. Some sociologists have estimated that at its peak the number of residents was closer to 200,000 (more than a third not listed on the lease).

The expansion of the CHA, along with urban renewal as a guise to salvage the city, is really a case study in the power of latent racism and government deceit and an example of a self-fulfilling prophecy of deterioration and disintegration. The majority of the housing complexes—the most extreme example was Robert Taylor Homes—are spread out along corridors of expressways that divided community areas into racially segregated districts. (Chicago is still referred to by many as the most segregated city in America.) Residents were trapped in enclaves without access to grocery and convenience stores but within walking distance to package liquor stores and currency exchanges. The "projects," outside those strictly for the elderly, provided ideal conditions for anomie and insurgency. Residents tended to be single women with two or more children. When the children became teenagers and young adults with poor primary education, they had few, if any, job opportunities. This environment was an ideal breeding ground for drugs, gangs, and violence. William Julius Wilson has written about these conditions in one of the major studies of modern urban sociology, *The Truly Disadvantaged: The Inner City, the Underclass, and Public Policy* (1987). By the start of the 1990s the political corruption and theft of resources had become so blatant that the federal agency Housing and Urban Development (HUD) moved in to run the CHA. In 2000 HUD introduced the Plan for Transformation, based on the principles of renewal of physical structures, the promotion of self-sufficiency, and the reform of the agency's administration.[1]

The Henry Horner Housing Project

Henry Horner Homes was located on a twenty-six-acre site on the Near West Side. Completed in 1957, it was named after the Illinois governor who held office from 1933 to 1940.[2] Besides being a five-minute drive or fifteen-minute walk from the medical center, it is a ten-minute train ride to the Loop. The project is located directly across from the United Center, home to the Bulls and the Blackhawks and a venue for big concerts. Henry Horner gained its notoriety when Alex Kotlowitz published his marvelous book, *There Are No Children Here: The Story of Two Boys Living in the Other America,* in 1992. In addition to describing the poignant struggles of Pharaoh and Lafayette (ages eight and ten, respectively), Kotlowitz vividly exposed the conditions of life in the other America. He identified the source of tension that seemed to engulf the Horner residents as being caused primarily by the gangs that were rampant in Chicago's housing projects. For example, in one week alone the police confiscated twenty-two guns and 330 grams of cocaine. But simply trying to live in a neighborhood that has become a black hole is unbearable in its own right. Kotlowitz described the living conditions—poor plumbing, elevators that didn't work, hallways without light, to mention only the most obvious—with clarity and a poetic style.

At the time I was reading the book I was also Rush's director of the Minority Medical Education Program, which had been conceptualized by the Association of American Medical Colleges and funded by the Robert Wood Johnson Foundation, with the goal of having three thousand underrepresented minority students enrolled in U.S. medical schools nationally by the year 2000. The thrust of the endeavor was to have a six-week prematriculation summer program (a head-start effort) for potential minority applicants to medical school. During that time I probably purchased as many as fifty copies of the book as a motivational force to keep the students' eyes on the prize of becoming a humanistic doctor. It eventually dawned on me that the same powerful social and ethical upheavals were highly relevant to members of RCSIP to whom I had also given copies of the book. I took the core group of student leaders to the top of the parking garage (my favorite observation deck) and pointed out Henry Horner Homes on the other side of the Eisenhower Expressway. I said, "There is the project described by Kotlowitz in his book. Don't you think we should try to do something to help the residents?"

On the basis of our discussion of the book, we contacted the Boys and Girls Club director at that time, Jerome Parham, who was very receptive to our proposal to start a tutoring program. Major Adams, a living legend at Horner, was director of the drum and bugle corps and had been instrumental in getting the hit musical group Earth, Wind, and Fire—all Horner kids—started. He was especially enthusiastic in his support of what we wanted to accomplish. He kept saying, "These kids really need this," and "No one really cares about them." The medical students were ecstatic when the Boys and Girls Club gave its consent for a group of predominantly white, middle-class medical students to begin tutoring and counseling inner-city black kids in the club's facility, located in the center of the housing project.

Safety again became a concern. I explained to the medical college administration that the Boys and Girls Club was a special sanctuary where no violence, drug transaction, or other unsavory behavior ever took place. In addition, there was a parking area next to the club so the RCSIP volunteers could enter and leave at a minute's notice. The other elements of maintaining safety—traveling in groups, casual dress, and the like—also applied. If for some reason medical students were stranded there, the car from Rush security could pick them up. Of course, we tried to avoid this as much as possible.

The tutoring sessions developed into close relationships between the RCSIP participants and the Horner kids, resulting in field trips to the zoo, which many had never seen; to a pizza parlor; and to the medical center as well as picnics in local parks. Some of the kids had rarely been outside the Horner complex before. Sitting down with a kid or a small group and going over math problems or simply reading to them is an effective mechanism for connecting. There was an intimacy there that didn't exist in the overcrowded and underfunded local public schools. Any potential racial overtones either didn't emerge or simply vanished. Major told me how much the Horner kids loved the students. "They really help," he said. Because of the positive effect the tutors were having, the mothers of the kids being tutored approached the medical students and asked for help with their number one health problem: childhood asthma. Just as I had predicted, the people of the community already knew what they needed.

Claudia and I spent a considerable amount of time meeting with community leaders to discuss the feasibility of an asthma control program. We met initially with Mamie Bone, the president of the Tenants' Advisory Council, whose main concern was having us establish a clinic at Horner. When we told her that was impossible, she became reluctant to accept our proposal and questioned our sincerity in trying to help. I felt she was reverting back to the myth that when it came to health care, the medical center wasn't interested.

But after many community meetings and discussions, the principal participants—Horner community leaders and Claudia and I as representatives of Rush with students often in attendance—came up with the idea that through cooperation by all parties, it would be possible to recruit, train, and place five local people to serve as community asthma workers (CAWs). To make the program complete, we would also approach all local health care providers in the area including Rush, the Mile Square Neighborhood Health Center, Cook

County (Stroger) and the University of Illinois hospitals, and the "Medicaid mills" on Madison Street, where asthmatic children frequently went for treatment. The CAWs would screen and identify asthmatic children, teach them to deal with their condition, find appropriate services for them, and follow them to be sure they were being properly cared for.

In the planning session, it was further agreed that the community would pick potential applicants for the positions, but we, as the health professionals, would make the final selection based on what we determined was required to function effectively in this newly devised position. The groundwork for a partnership had been laid. With the help of the students and Rush faculty specializing in childhood asthma—Dr. James Moy from Rush and Cook County and Dr. Evelyn Grant from Rush pediatrics and immunology—we would train and monitor the CAWs.

The selection process was quite an education in itself. We had the students interview all the applicants first. The students got to meet a wide spectrum of Horner residents, mostly women, and learned about their backgrounds. The students were exposed to the effects of addiction, prison, and abuse and the incredible struggle required simply to survive and protect their children from a life of segregation, racism, violence, and self-destruction.

Here are two examples from the interviewing: When asked what she had been doing, one young woman keeping repeating, "I've been away." Finally, she admitted she had been in prison and rolled up her sleeve to show the needle marks from her heroin addiction. In answer to why he was sure he could become an asthma worker, one of the few male applicants said, "Because I'm like Mike." When he finally recognized that the students didn't get it, he put on his "shades" and explained, "I look just like Michael Jordan."

Five African American women ranging in age from their midtwenties to their late thirties, all with high school diplomas and one with some college, were chosen. Three of the women had lived in Henry Horner all their lives, the other two for more than ten years each. The initial training consisted of a series of interrelated stages that were taught over an intense two-week period (thirty hours in all); although ambitious, we took care to keep it from being burdensome or stressful. The CAWs were first given a thorough schooling in the basic concepts, facts, and terms necessary for a fundamental understanding of the ailment. Short quizzes, oral and multiple-choice exams, and classroom discussions were used as formative evaluation. The medical students, who helped write the training protocols, were invaluable in all these sessions. It was quite an enlightening experience for them and broke down any misconceptions they had about the local women's ability to learn the material. In turn, "the asthma ladies" showed love and respect for their student partners. Such relationships are invaluable; they are a vivid example that shared goals transcend race, social status, and geographical boundaries.

The following phase of the training focused on the more strictly medical aspects of asthma, including the application of treatment modalities such as how to use metered-dose inhalers, spacers, nebulizers, and peak-flow meters, and the importance of having a plan of action. The CAWs were also made familiar with the different types of medications used in treating asthma as well as the role the physical environment plays in triggering attacks. They learned how to "desensitize" a room by changing elements of the physical environment (shag rugs, cats) that act as triggers. These medical care skills and procedures were taught jointly by the physicians and the medical students in a series of lectures and hands-on demonstrations.

In conjunction with the medical training, the CAWs were taught the fundamental principles of case management and family advocacy by Jackie U'Dean, director of children's support services, who was program coordinator for a large-scale asthma control program at La Rabida Children's Hospital, an affiliate of the University of Chicago. Following this first training phase, the CAWS were taught how to establish and maintain an effective intervention—a very sophisticated concept and activity. Role-playing with immediate feedback was used in these training sessions. The CAWs were also taught how to collect data, since it was needed for evaluation and was essential for keeping the program going. The medical students learned as much, if not more, than they taught. The closeness between them and the CAWs became evident by the end of the training period. Since all the CAWs were on welfare and because RCSIP did not have the funds to actually employ them at least at a compensatory level, they were paid for their work through honoraria, which, at that time, would not affect their government benefits. (This changed with the Clinton administration's Welfare to Work initiative.) The full extent of training lasted about two months.

The real test of the training phase was whether local residents could be trained as competent community outreach workers capable of finding, teaching, and monitoring inner-city children who were suffering from asthma and keeping their symptoms under control. We had a small graduation ceremony followed by a lunch at the CAWs favorite Italian restaurant. The CAWs were ready, and we all knew it.

Some of the asthmatic children who were discovered through the program lived in chaotic, dysfunctional households: parents and guardians on drugs, relatives and other adults and children moving in and out of the home, supervision left to grandparents or foster families, and such poverty and deprivation that neighborhood pantries and shelters became a major source of food and clothing. Death, serious illness, and violence played an inordinate role in the already overstressed lives of many of these children. Finding and following the asthmatic children was not easy, even for seasoned project dwellers like the CAWs. For two-thirds of the fifteen children initially enrolled in the program, their last visit to a doctor had been at the emergency room of Cook County Hospital. The influence of this and related circumstances had an overwhelming effect on the students. Through the CAWs' efforts to reach and help families with asthmatic children, the medical students were exposed to a social gradient that existed in Horner just as in any other social aggregate. In other words, some families were simply worse off than others and lacked any discernible social support and little control over their lives.

In this regard, the CAWs became deeply involved with the lives of their children's families. For example, they got a drug-addicted mother into rehabilitation, they found legal help for a parent who was having difficulties with the Department of Children and Family Services, they encouraged a pregnant parent to seek prenatal care, they located food and clothing for a destitute family, and they assisted in funeral arrangements for a mother who died. Too often politicians, bureaucrats, social researchers, and theorists bandy about notions concerning the plight of the poor and the disadvantaged without having any firsthand experience with the complexity of their lives and their prospects for improving them. The RCSIP students were exposed to the living conditions and ubiquitous stress that pervade this kind of physical and social environment. One student put it eloquently:

> This experience had a profound effect on me. I think it changed my life. Actually, I don't know how to describe it. Here are these five women. All of them have children. One of them has seven. But they are such loving mothers—they are so considerate. They are so wise. They are angry with the insensitivity of society toward them (they have every right to be)—lack of health care, insensitive doctors, all that stuff. But they weren't hostile toward us! In fact they were kind and considerate. They were like our teachers, explaining things to us, describing what life is like in the projects. When I got home I called my mother. I told her I thought I knew something about how poor people survive in the projects, but I knew nothing. They are loving mothers who need a chance. How fortunate we are. How fortunate I am to get to know them. I hope I can help them in some way.

Because of the stressful and turbulent environment of life in the projects, we anticipated that some staff turnover was bound to take place. In fact, it happened before the end of the first full year of operation. Given the opportunity, one woman was able to move out of Horner; another was recruited by Oprah, who was filming a TV version of *There Are No Children Here*. Because of the prestige associated with being one of the CAWs, it was possible to find and quickly train two new members, who were supervised by the other CAWs. The trained had become trainers. Over the remaining years of operation, however, there was very little turnover of the program staff.

With all these extra challenges it was unrealistic to assume that each worker could handle ten cases. At the end of the first year, with only three CAWs working, they had enrolled twenty-six asthmatic children into the program, of which twenty were still actively involved. Reasons for dropping out included moving away (buildings were being torn down), death in the extended family, and dysfunctional families (drug abuse, disintegration), but rarely lack of interest. As soon as the two new CAWs were out in the field five more children were added to the program. The number of children enrolled in the program peaked at about fifty, and for those who remained active, there was a consistent pattern of success.

If finding, monitoring, and controlling the entire population of asthmatic children in Horner was an impossible goal, there were, nonetheless, other achievable interventions that allowed the community to play a significant role in confronting the ailment. Almost every family had very little, if any, factual information about the probable sources, treatment, and duration of asthma in young children. It seemed as if about half the parents or guardians believed that their children would outgrow asthma by the time they were teenagers or young adults. The other half believed that children with asthma could not, under any circumstances, engage in any serious physical activity, such as sports. There was also a basic lack of knowledge among several of the physicians with offices on the Near West Side, one of whom had actually decided that the children were not asthmatic and would prescribe cough medicine to treat them. Ignorance about the condition and how it affected children still existed, despite the finding that almost all the adults had supposedly received some instruction from their children's own doctor.

The CAWs were magnificent in getting the message out to the community about asthma and what the residents' responsibilities were regarding care of the children. They also went to the schools and talked to the principals and teachers about the program and how they could use the services of the CAWs. They even took their asthmatic charges to see their doctors or nurse practitioners, who soon realized what an asset these workers were in keeping the children's condition under control.

With the assistance of the medical students, the CAWs held community meetings at the Boys and Girls Club, usually around some special occasion such as Halloween, with food, balloons, and prizes for the kids. During these events they talked freely about the seriousness of asthma and answered questions. Starting in the third year, the students and CAWs ran a three-day camping experience in a forest preserve at which about one-third of the kids who showed up weren't even asthmatic. The goal was to show that asthmatic kids could enjoy the outdoors just like everyone else. For the CAWs their identity gave them a great deal of respect from their neighbors and the community at large. Moreover, they exuded a new self-respect, a sense of Jesse Jackson's motto "I am somebody." They had clearly shown that they could learn and apply sophisticated medical knowledge and skills and, in the act of caring, felt the fulfillment of helping people, not only the children but also their families, in a compassionate and humane manner. Their new identity came from their actions.

For the medical students, being actively involved at Horner fostered empathy toward the residents and the kind of life they had to live. Even though they were primarily committed to establishing a community program in the control of childhood asthma, the students became aware that there were other pertinent and all-encompassing issues that permeated life in Horner. This important insight contributed greatly to the significance of the experience. For example, the willingness of the community leaders to share these problems is an excellent indication of the trust they had in the students personally and as representatives of Rush. Such social awareness is essential to any real reform or change. As Goulet (1971) has pointed out, "Development . . . involves human attitudes and preferences, self-defined goals, and criteria for determining what is the tolerable cost to be borne in the course of change" (35). Fundamentally, these are far more important than better resource allocation, upgraded skills, or the rationalization of administrative procedures. Unless these "technical" components are accepted by the community as being good, they soon lose their effectiveness in the course of daily life.

As part of my assessment of program efficacy (Eckenfels 1994) I made a concerted effort to interview key community representatives about this relationship. In consultation with the CAWs, I selected five people who were not only revered by the community but also had spent a considerable number of years working or living there. The list included the director of the Boys and Girls Club, a police officer who had spent more than twenty years watching over the local residents, the head of the Residents' Advisory Council, a community activist with a city-wide reputation, and the director of a men's organization dedicated to getting the young men living in Horner to take a socially responsible stance in dealing with gangs and drugs.

Since I had five years of experience in survey research at the National Opinion Research Center at the University of Chicago, was trained in participant-observer techniques, and used these techniques extensively in my community work in Mississippi and Mile Square (where Horner is located), I was able to develop an interview schedule that allowed me to spend at least one hour talking with each of the five respondents. The interviews—all open ended but following a carefully designed set of questions—revealed very similar outcomes. The interviewees all raved about how important the asthma project was to the community. They emphasized that not only were the CAWs helping asthmatic kids, but the establishment of the project in the community had made the residents aware of the disease and what was needed to control it. As one respondent put it, "We knew there was a lot of asthma, but we didn't know how to control it." Here are some examples of other responses:

> "Seeing those women, the asthma ladies, looking after those kids made us all proud."
>
> "Getting rid of shag rugs, old cat [things], and stuff like that really makes a difference in helping [the children] breathe."
>
> "Having picnics and a camp and getting those kids out of Horner into the fresh air had never been done before."
>
> "We are so pleased that Pres [Rush–Presbyterian–St. Luke's Medical Center] is involved. It ain't that we don't love County [Cook County Hospital], but to have the other hospital's help really is important, and those medical students really are good—God musta sent them."

These testimonies offered high praise of the program and its impact on the community. There was another recurrent outcome from the interviews. In each instance, the community representatives offered their perspective on the community's two major concerns: violence and drugs. My respondents reported that since Henry Horner is located directly across the street from the United Center, where the Chicago Bulls and Blackhawks play, it was an ideal place for suburban and North Side fans to pick up their drugs of choice, namely, cocaine and marijuana, before or after a game. A common refrain was that, in the days of Michael Jordan, the closer the Bulls got to winning the NBA championship, the greater the quantity of drugs being sold. The drug business was managed by two different gangs that on occasion battled over control of the territory. Levitt and Dubner's (2005) analysis of gangs corresponds to the situation we observed in Henry Horner. The gang battles were franchise fights for control of the local territory, and the "dealers" were the street soldiers, who, incidentally, did indeed live with their moms. The African American police officer whose main beat was the Boys and Girls Club related the following story:

> I've been to over thirty funerals of kids killed in gang wars. Not too long ago, there was a big gang fight just outside the club. I saw a kid I knew shoot and kill another kid, who I also knew. After the police and ambulance came (I called them), in a moment of despair, I asked two boys, about ten or twelve, who were shooting pool, what they thought would happen if we could get rid of all the drugs in Horner. Their response was, "We be poor."

There is more to this story than simply an interesting digression. The medical students had acquired a good understanding of why "project people" distrusted the authority inherent in what they referred to as "the system." The residents believed that the city (the mayor, the police chief, the fire fighters, the cops with the flak jackets) allowed the drug trade to go on because it was such a moneymaker and catered to the pleasure of members of the white middle class who could afford the price of season tickets to see their favorite superstars. Incidentally, on special occasions, a few of the Bulls did visit the Boys and Girls Club, giving the kids sneakers and jerseys and, at least once that I know of, serving food at the annual Thanksgiving dinner.

Each program has at least one experience that leaves an indelible mark. I would like to end the Horner story with two personal anecdotes. As I have pointed out, directly across from Horner on Wood Street is the United Center, where the Bulls and Blackhawks play. The new facility, built between 1992 and 1994, is considered one of the largest and most modern arenas in the country. Prior to construction of the building, the six-acre area housed the old Chicago Stadium, which was imploded in 1994 a few months before the official opening of the new arena. I remember visiting Horner on a hot and exceptionally humid August afternoon following the day of the implosion. The little grass that was in the grounds surrounding Horner had vanished in the heat, leaving dust that blew in waves across the landscape. A few short blocks away, workers were renovating the Lake Street Elevated, another source of dirt and debris. But the most distressing sight was the huge, thick cloud of dust generated by the implosion that hung over Horner, choking asthmatic kids with watery eyes and overworked lungs simply trying to breathe. No one knew or cared.

Shortly after the United Center was completed and just before it would officially open in the fall of 1994, the groundskeepers decided to test the sprinkler system. (Much of this area was later converted to additional parking space.)

Keep in mind that this new complex, with its perfectly manicured grounds and gorgeous green grass, was directly across the street from the housing project. When the sprinklers were turned on, Horner kids poured across Wood Street, climbed the fence surrounding the center, and headed for the geysers of cool, fresh, clear water. Before they had gone twenty yards the entrance doors of the magnificent center, radiating like Oz in the sun, seemed to open automatically, and security guards with raised nightsticks (most of them black) began running toward the youngsters. The children stopped dead in their tracks, quickly recognized what they were up against, turned 180 degrees, and went back to where they belonged.

The situation in Horner is a revelation of the enormity of the challenges that must be faced in trying to reach a community that has been alienated from the larger society. This observation is not meant to imply that poor, inner-city populations cannot be helped, but, rather, that only by making a proposed intervention part of the social fabric of the community residents' lives can the intervention become viable. In short, there is more to fostering a life worth living than changes in lifestyles proposed by well-intended outsiders. The typical attitude that surrounds notions about poor and disadvantaged communities, about what their needs are and how best to meet those needs, leaves out the real source of expertise—the community—and what it has to offer in finding solutions. It is not only needs assessments that lead to solutions; resource assessments really count.

Casa Guatemala

Casa Guatemala is located in Uptown, a community area six miles north of the Loop. Uptown has an interesting history, but its growth and decline follow a pattern similar to that of other community areas in Chicago. In the first quarter of the twentieth century it experienced a commercial boom. It had ballrooms, theaters, and even a movie studio along its main drag, Broadway. Like so many Chicago communities, Uptown's fortunes changed during the Great Depression. By the end of World War II living conditions had worsened, and former luxury apartments were subdivided. Because landlords didn't require long-term leases or security deposits, Uptown became a haven to recent migrants and Chicago's poor. In the 1950s whites from Appalachia; Japanese Americans from California; and Native Americans from Wisconsin, Minnesota, and Oklahoma settled in Uptown's affordable but deteriorating housing. The American Indian Center in Chicago, the oldest and largest urban Native American center in the country, is located in Uptown. Temporary worker offices exist where mostly men can be hired by the day to do jobs that are dirty and require hard physical labor. There are also a number of halfway houses for addicts and people diagnosed with mental illness.

When I was a student at the University of Chicago in the early 1960s, we went to Uptown to hear "authentic" bluegrass music. To forestall bar fights with broken bottles and glasses, beer was served in plastic cups. Beginning in the 1960s a new flow of immigrants took refuge in Uptown. Sephardic Jews from Eastern Europe; political refugees from Central America; and families escaping from Vietnam, Thailand, and Cambodia turned Uptown into an even more amazing cultural mix. They brought with them their languages, their cuisines, their health needs, and most of all their aspirations. In my community health course I would send some of the students to the public health clinic to see firsthand the health problems of recent arrivals. I recall the students being overwhelmed by the variety of parasites found in the Jewish immigrants from Russia. Although many community initiatives (such as Model Cities, Heart of Uptown Coalition) have had a revitalizing effect on Uptown, the neighborhood is far from an ideal "melting pot." In 2000, one-third of the population of 63,551 was foreign born.

The first wave of Guatemalans to Chicago came prior to the 1980s. They were intellectuals, union organizers, students, and activists who had fled the violent civil war. They were initially provided sanctuary in Catholic churches and taken into their parishes. In the early 1990s the U.S.-based sanctuary movement offered them critical protection from Guatemalan-based death squads. The Chicago Religious Task Force created an "underground railroad," bringing other displaced Guatemalans from Arizona to Chicago. The second wave came in the mid-1990s, and the 2000 census reported that there were 19,444 Guatemalans living in metropolitan Chicago. Fear of drawing Immigration and Naturalization Service (INS) attention led the new immigrants to disperse to other communities farther west, such as Elgin. There is a tendency to lump Guatemalans with other Latino groups in Chicago. The majority of the more recent Guatemalan immigrants are Mayan campesinos and often have little or no formal education and work primarily in the city's restaurants and factories or in the suburbs as gardeners and domestic workers.

Since its inception in 1986, Casa Guatemala has sought to create a haven for Guatemalans and other Latin Americans who have immigrated to this country in search of a sanctuary from political turmoil, war, and economic disintegration. The motto of Casa Guatemala, *Nuestro compromiso son nuestras comunidades,* roughly translated as "Our commitment reflects the most basic necessities in our community," aptly states the principles on which the organization was created. The actual community center facility was located in an old office building on Wilson Avenue. Mayan heritage is very important to the new

immigrants' sense of self and community. The Mayan people have been colo-
nized and enslaved for more than five hundred years in the name of European
exploration. The organizers of Casa Guatemala are sensitive to the problem of
desplazamiento, or "displacement" (to be removed from one's space or home).
The situation was further exacerbated by the growing intensity of the civil war,
which had started in 1954. By the 1970s, more than 450 villages had been
destroyed and two hundred thousand residents had left the country. The services provided by Casa Guatemala—immigrant referrals, legal counseling, and
lessons in English as a second language—were crucial to the new arrivals' sur-
vival and adaptation.

RCSIP was introduced to Casa Guatemala, as it was to other grassroots
community organizations, through the former's reputation and through personal contact. A young physician from Argentina, Veronica Plaza, who was
doing graduate work in biochemistry at Rush, had been volunteering at the
community center and, when she heard of RCSIP, sought me out. She explained
the plight of recent immigrants and their status as political refugees to Claudia
and me along with a group of students. As the word got out among other RCSIP
members, two medical students already fluent in Spanish came forward to participate. They wanted to help in any way that might be useful. One of them had
been a Spanish major in college; she soon found out that her smooth Castilian
speech didn't register that easily with those from a strong Mayan cultural background. Nonetheless, the community center administration and the people
who used the facility as a commons were warm, friendly, and accepting toward
the students. Every time any of us visited Casa Guatemala we were fed indigenous food, particularly *moloch,* a combination of spices, herbs, and pork or
chicken, in a tortilla shell. The food, like everything else they offered, came
from the heart. The students loved Casa Guatemala and Casa Guatemala loved
them.

Veronica had recruited a young Rush fellow in internal medicine, who was
also of Latino heritage, to start a simple health assessment two nights a week.
The team of two doctors and two students were struck by the fact that for many
of the people who showed up, it was their first examination by a physician
since they had arrived in Chicago, in some cases, years ago. To try to find
answers for why this was the case, we decided to conduct a brief survey to learn
some basic sociodemographic information, which included a self-assessment
of health status. Under my guidance, the Spanish-speaking students devised a
short questionnaire that the respondents could understand. The findings were
startling in two ways: respondents had no idea of where to go to seek health
care, and they were afraid of drawing INS attention and being deported if they

went to any agency that had government affiliation, such as a public health clinic. Those who had ventured to some of the existing clinics said they were mistreated and not understood. They felt shamed by their ignorance.

Even cursory physicals and histories revealed the usual culprits—high blood pressure, diabetes, and parasites—all ailments that can be treated or controlled. Most of the people participating in the health screening were women and children. Less than one in ten of the adults spoke even rudimentary English. In almost every case, birth control was out of the question. There was a strong sense of family, especially among those who were separated from their loved ones back in Guatemala. Another matter that emerged from the assessment was fear, even in the United States, of some kind of retaliation by the Guatemalan military police, some of whom were being trained in assault tactics at Fort Benning, Georgia. But access to health care remained the major barrier. There was not only the inability to find health care settings that were receptive to the new arrivals, but also the bewilderment of the Guatemalan people about how to take advantage of existing facilities.

We were stymied about what to do next; after much internal discussion, the health care team decided that the most immediate and best thing we could offer was more thorough health assessments for as many people as we could reach. The center staff agreed. The format was a three-day extensive health evaluation conducted at Casa Guatemala. With Veronica's assistance we were able to recruit another eight physicians, and using the St. Basil vertical and horizontal integration model, the team performed an extensive health evaluation of more than two hundred people, including about fifty men, of all ages during one of Chicago's worst heat waves (temperatures above one hundred for more than a week). The patients, ranging from newborns to the very elderly, rotated through numbered stations for different procedures—taking blood pressures, drawing blood, screening for neurological signs—so the procession of people being evaluated flowed smoothly. Brochures and other materials, including advice on birth control methods, written in Spanish were available. The screening took place in a huge empty loft above the community center. Large industrial fans were placed at each end of the room in an unsuccessful attempt to cool the place; they simply redistributed the hot air. It was quite a sight watching the team work. Dressed in their surgical greens to keep cool, wiping the sweat from their eyes, shouting orders back and forth, and requesting more of this and help with that, they exuded an enthusiasm and purpose that permeated the atmosphere. Like the doctors, the senior and junior medical students did medical evaluations; the preclinical students drew blood, took blood pressures, and performed typical triage procedures. A referral system was set up to get the seriously ill to clinics or hospitals. More than one person was taken to an emergency room suffering from severe dehydration.

At the end of three days, we reflected on what we had done. First and foremost, we had provided health care, regardless of how limited and singular, to people who had had none. As a result of all the preliminary actions leading up to the health evaluations, we were closer to understanding the culture and social status of Guatemalans in Chicago. On the basis of the data and, more important, the humanity of the people served, we were able to formulate a strategy to help them. Using the health evaluations along with the survey data, we developed a mechanism to overcome bureaucratic obstacles and get the people enrolled in Health Department clinics for much-needed medical services. We contacted the director of programs for Hispanics at the Chicago Department of Health, who committed herself to work with us, especially regarding the public health clinic in Uptown. We also visited all the Uptown community organizations and social service agencies to get their assistance. The medical students initially accompanied some of the most apprehensive people on their first clinic visit. Because of their strong Mayan heritage, many still felt uncomfortable. The CommunityHealth clinic (see chapter 2), with its large Latino base, accepted patients immediately. Since the students were familiar with how CommunityHealth functions, it made the transition less traumatic. It was still quite a distance (two buses if you don't go by car), but it was a place where the Guatemalans were openly welcomed.

RCSIP had been accepted as a real partner by Casa Guatemala. It was a joy to visit. The students were becoming very familiar with Mayan culture, including certain religious practices. I had the privilege of presenting the survey data and health evaluations at a symposium on Latin American human rights held at the University of Chicago in 1995. When it came time for me to speak I introduced myself as the token gringo on the panel, which got a roar from the audience and a standing ovation from my Guatemalan friends. By and large our work at Casa Guatemala was over now. As a fitting close, the RCSIP participants were invited to a banquet celebrating Central American independence on September 15, 1996. Besides the incredible native Mayan food, there was handwoven Mayan clothing on sale. The students were attracted to the colorful blouses, belts, and vests. I was given a special award, in the form of a diploma, for "devoting his time and efforts in behalf of our organization and the Guatemalan people."

Occasionally, my wife and I were invited to certain events. At one that I will never forget we heard Juan Gerardi, the auxiliary bishop of Guatemala City, speak on the poverty, deprivation, and lack of social justice that engulfed his country. His words echoed the liberation theology—the relationship between Roman Catholicism and political activism particularly in areas of social justice, poverty, and human rights—of the dedicated clergy who put themselves on the line to fight political oppression throughout Central America. On April 26, 1998, after releasing a church report on the country's civil war, which had ended in December 1996, he was murdered.[3] As I reflected on this, I thought of our lack of awareness in this country that thirteen hundred women in Guatemala have been killed since 2001 or that the struggle by the indigenous Campesino, Union, and Popular Movement (MISCP) continues against the ratification of the Central American Free Trade Agreement (CAFTA), which perpetuates sweatshop wages and slave labor practices. An awareness of these struggles has added social and political dimensions to the students' perspective as future health providers.

Chapter 5

The Community Today, Tomorrow the World

Public health is a subject about which one country can learn from another.

—Amartya Sen, "Passage to China"

There's no place on earth like the world.

—Brendan Behan, *The Hostage*

In the 1990s the United States, like the rest of the industrialized world, was going global, and cultural diversity was becoming the norm. The new global perspective was finding its way into health care and medicine: The AIDS pandemic does not stop at the border; people carrying contagious diseases can be in a country thousands of miles away in ten hours. The potential of telemedicine for transmitting medical information via computer networks was emerging. There was a new spirit of cooperation among scientists and clinicians worldwide. And there was already a group, Médecins sans frontières, or Doctors without Borders, dedicated to going to the poorest and most remote regions of the world to aid the sick and suffering.[1] In the early 1990s, universal rights to health and well-being were getting revived attention at home, especially since the United States was, and still is, the only industrialized country in the world without universal health care. This sudden interest in international health added a new dimension to my focus on active participation in health care reform. Besides the obvious medical implication, such reforms now had a powerful political and social aspect not only on a local and national level, but internationally as well.

I was also becoming more personally involved in international health. During a summer visit to Rush, Professor Jeffrey Levett, an old friend and a professor at the National School of Public Health in Athens, Greece, stirred my interest in the emerging challenges of a global perspective in health and illness. He persuaded me that globalization provided an opportunity to get health care professionals from many countries to cooperate on addressing health issues that affected all of us. Moreover, the focus on the economic outcomes of globalization through such efforts as the North American Free Trade Agreement (NAFTA) glossed over the horrific deprivation and political oppression of the poorer nations. He invited me to give a presentation on health manpower development in the United States at the second annual meeting of the Federation of International Cooperation of Health Services and Systems Research Centers (FICOSSER) in Delphi, Greece, in May 1996. On the basis of that presentation, I was invited to Belgrade, Serbia, by Dr. Momčilo Babič, director of Bezanijska kosa Medical Center, where I began working with a group of progressive physicians with a strong public health point of view. I eventually became a member of the European Center for Peace and Development, an agency of the United Nations. Under the auspices of that organization I participated in an international conference on public health and peace in Skopje, Macedonia, in December 2001. Professor Levett and I coined the phrase (which later became the theme of the conference) "The health of the public is a catalyst for peace and development." The subject of international health was becoming a major part of my life, and I wanted to use my commitment to support students who had a desire to serve abroad.

All the while students were helping refugees in Chicago they were also interested in helping vulnerable and disenfranchised people in the Third World. The seed was planted early when those who had gone abroad relayed their experiences to fellow students. Not only were these experiences exciting, they were enlightening as well. As one student put it, they opened your eyes to a totally different culture where health and illness take on a different meaning; the effect is so profound, it changes you for life.

In my discussions with medical students who were seriously interested, we began devising a way for promoting student involvement in international health. The students decided to set up a new program, the Rush Students for International Health and Medicine (RSIHM), which was actually a logical spin-off from RCSIP. As with RSCIP, the aim was to have RSIHM become a full-scale program in its own right. The creation of such an organization was inevitable. Because of my own interest, I became more of a partner than an advisor. My responsibility was to develop a framework that could be used to validate the significance of involving students (even for a short time) in poor and developing countries as an adjunct to their education as future physicians.

I turned to the work of Martha Nussbaum, the University of Chicago's Ernst Freund Professor of Law and Ethics, for insights.[2] The foundation of the truly participatory process, according to Nussbaum (1997b), incorporates three core values: critical self-examination, the ideal of a world citizen, and the development of the narrative imagination. Nussbaum advocates a close scrutiny of cultural traditions. "A truly Socratic education," she writes, "should be suited to the pupils' circumstances and context and concerned with a variety of different norms and traditions." She draws upon the Stoics and their philosophy of the "citizen of the world," which holds that self-knowledge is enhanced by knowledge of others and that problems are better solved "if we face them in the broader context, our imaginations unconstrained by narrow partisanship" (14). I felt that in a global world, to paraphrase Nussbaum, the contemporary medical practitioner must become a citizen-physician for social justice.

The students found the ideal of world citizenship particularly relevant for the education and practice of physicians in the twenty-first century. I pointed out, as a method of reinforcing their conviction, that the modern physician cannot avoid feeling the impact of this worldview even if he or she does not embrace the idea. Simply to function adequately as a health care giver in the present-day multicultural environment, one has to know something about what people from other cultures are like. Moreover, as Nussbaum makes clear, "it is morally good to learn about others and to understand where they are coming from." A truly professional education, therefore, provides such a perspective as an integral part of the personal learning and development of the prospective physician.

This conceptual framework gave us the theoretical underpinnings we were looking for. Not only was the motivation present but, as was evident from the students' actions in RCSIP, the confidence to be able to form an international health program was there also. In other words, since they had demonstrated that they could devise, organize, and sustain a series of community service projects, they felt confident they could broaden their outlook as well. As expected, the students made no small plans.

From planning for RCSIP, they knew their first job was developing a rationale for the program that would be acceptable to the medical school administration. Collectively, we teased out a number of components that gave the idea credence. Since Chicago is one of the most culturally diverse cities in the United States, firsthand experience in the countries of origin of many of its recent arrivals provides an avenue to the roots of cultural diversity—an important factor in the care and treatment of members of those various ethnic groups. Experience in other countries also gives students an actual basis for cultural comparisons of norms, beliefs, and behaviors and their implications for perceived states of health and illness, thus allowing for a better understanding of similarities and differences and identifying strengths and weaknesses when it comes to how health care is delivered. Fundamentally, an international health perspective is essential if the world is to survive in the new millennium when AIDS, malaria, tuberculosis, and other communicable diseases are on a rampage. Such a perspective embodies environmental, social, economic, and political factors. Exposure to other societies alerts students to the interrelationship of these factors. When you have an opportunity to see foreigners in the light of the countries and cultures of their origin, you acquire a sensitivity that simply can't be gained from seeing them here. Furthermore, it is the moral and social responsibility of health professionals in developed nations, especially the United States, with its advanced medical science and technology, to cooperate through joint ventures, exchange programs, and resource dispersion with less fortunate countries.

Working abroad allows students to engage in such cooperative ventures. An open exchange program (involving students, clinicians, researchers, teachers) with other countries allows everyone to learn from each other through reciprocity. Collaboration, whether in research, education, or patient care, leads to understanding and solutions of common problems through discovery and application. Using our technical expertise to help other less fortunate countries with limited resources, especially the developing and marginal nations, allows us to make a direct contribution to their medical practice. In return, they can show us how they continue to provide health care without this technology. As Dostoevsky has proclaimed, "We are all responsible for all." Finally, it was my contention that students exposed to this process will learn the subtleties of open and trusting interaction, that is, how to avoid paternalism and the "know it all" attitude that Americans seem to project the world over.

In 1997, building on these propositions, the students developed the following mission statement:

> As students in medical school nearing the end of the century, we are in a prime position to participate in changing the health care milieu. Whereas the four basic tenets of medicine have always been promotion, prevention, care, and cure, it seems as if the primary focus has been given to care and cure. Now we are looking more to disease prevention and health promotion as the means to achieve a state of well-being. But these are broad-scope concepts, and, in that respect, we must look at health as a global phenomenon if promotion and prevention are to be truly understood. What affects one country affects all, and, as we have seen, an outbreak of tuberculosis in Central America and the Caribbean can easily spread to their North American neighbors. The pandemic of AIDS throughout Africa offers even stronger evidence of what can happen and [of] the fact that none of us, especially those in the health professions, are immune to risk at a global level.

As American medical students being prepared to face the diseases and illnesses of the twenty-first century, we need international health experiences to understand the culturally diverse societies in which physicians are practicing medicine. The international health experience allows us to provide services to underserved populations while relying upon our history taking and physical diagnosis skills as the main means for providing these services. The cultural context in which these fundamental medical procedures take place provides an awareness that makes us sensitive to all the patients we serve throughout our careers. Not only will the foreign communities where we offer our services benefit, but also the different communities where we practice in the United States will reap these newly acquired skills and benefits as well. We see these endeavors as learning through service.

It was agreed that RSIHM should be established on the same principles as RCSIP, namely, that it should be student run, voluntary, and self-perpetuating. In short, students should make every effort to keep RSIHM out of the control of the medical school administration to avoid losing its spontaneity and originality.

Following this line of reasoning, a short list of achievable goals and objectives for presentation to the medical college administration was prepared. The goals were to provide students with experiences in developing countries as a way of broadening their knowledge and humanism, to expose them to different cultures as a way of improving their understanding of cultural diversity in our own society, and to create a self-perpetuating and sustainable program of international health. The objectives were to provide a continuity of international health experiences for Rush students beginning in their M1 year; to maintain an organization that is both initiated and run by students and is effective in terms of breadth of experiences, detailed reports, and systematic evaluation; to acquire the funding and resources necessary to keep the program going; and to have RSIHM become an integral component of the medical college.

As with RCSIP, certain components had to be in place prior to instituting the program. The first was a survey as a mechanism for the recruitment of faculty with international contacts. Dr. Donna Bergen, a neurologist with a strong interest in international health, had conducted a survey of faculty already involved in international health, and we used her data as a resource for recruitment. With Dr. Bergen's list, we hosted a luncheon that resulted in finding twenty faculty members who were willing to sponsor the students in countries where they had contacts.

The second was the collection and organization of existing information and data pertaining to international health, with special emphasis on education and application (experiential learning). On the basis of these data we were able to create an organizational scheme that could serve as a cross-reference of (1) individuals, including Rush faculty, friends, and other contacts; (2) organizations, such as International Health and Medical Education Consortium, the U.S. Agency for International Development (USAID), Doctors without Borders, embassies, and physicians' groups; (3) programs involving training, intervention, and assessment; and (4) funding sources, whether philanthropic, institutional, or governmental. A resource library with reference materials of a cultural and historical nature was also created.

The students developed a protocol for orientation, participation, and assessment that would not be limited to immunizations and safety checks but would include cultural sensitivity and political awareness. Travel arrangements required obtaining not only round-trip air travel between Chicago and the destination, but also a description of who would meet the student, how they would get to and from the site, and what to expect regarding living conditions. The key element to the success of the program was determining what was expected of the student participant. Just as in RCSIP we had the goal of finding a way to get students out of the academic health center and into the "real world" by immersing them in poor, disadvantaged, and culturally diversified communities, we promoted the same approach in the international health sphere. London and Paris were not sites we were looking for.

In addition, RSIHM had to address some obstacles bigger than the ones faced by RCSIP when it began. For starters, acquiring funding for student international health activities is extremely difficult because it is so expensive. International agencies and nongovernmental organizations (NGOs) have limited funds, and keeping their projects operating with full-time skilled professionals takes precedence over everything else. The immediate available source of funding was summer research fellowships from the dean's office. But for a number of reasons, it was almost impossible to formulate proposals for going to a developing country that fit a rigid research protocol: first, the students knew very little about the countries they were going to; second, time constraints limited any systematic epidemiology studies; and, third, the students could not yet understand the taboos and restrictions of the cultures in which they would be working. Without such awareness they could do more harm than good. What they could do, however, is observe, listen, interact, reflect, and grow and develop. From my perspective, their basic "method of investigation" was keeping a journal and logbook. Because of my training in social research, I was able to provide them with the rudimentary methods of ethnography and suggest that they learn to relate what they experience "there" with what they experience "here." Moreover, it is during and after the international health experiences that the students begin to understand and focus on what they have gained.

Both Rob McKersie, who writes about his experiences in his book *In the Foothills of Medicine* (2005), and Geeta Maker, a recognized activist at St. Basil's, eloquently project the power of personal experiences in the developing world. Rob began his international health work in South Africa:

> I had the good fortune of being awarded a Dean's Scholarship for the summer between my first and second year of medical school to work in Alexandria, South Africa. I volunteered for six weeks in a clinic that was on the edge of one of the largest "shantytowns" in South Africa. My duties during this time were varied. I worked in all departments of the clinic [and participated] in many health outreach programs into the neighboring shantytown. I even did a rotation in South Africa's famous Baragwanna Hospital, which resides right next to Soweto, South Africa. This is the world's largest public hospital and with it came the eye-opening realization of the dramatic needs of the underserved in this world.
>
> My medical experience in Africa was the spark that has driven my volunteer international medical work to date. The poverty and need that I witnessed in South Africa was unspeakable. My desire to help alleviate some of these inequities in the world has been the reason I have subsequently volunteered roughly every eighteen months in developing countries with Nepal being the country that I have volunteered in the most. Rush Students for International Health and Medicine (RSIHM) laid the groundwork for my continual medical work in other countries, work that will go on throughout the rest of my life.
>
> My work in South Africa and more recently in Nepal has taught me invaluable clinical skills. In these countries, where medical supplies are scarce, medical professionals are forced to develop and use their clinical diagnostic skills to a higher degree than their counterparts in more developed countries—especially medical professionals who have access to diagnostic laboratories or high-tech imaging devices like those we have in the United States.
>
> Finally, RSIHM taught me the important lesson that the world is one community, that I, a family doctor on the south side of Chicago, can make an important contribution not only to the health care of my patients in Chicago, but also to the people of the world. This international

volunteerism is vitally important, not only for the actual physical health of our international citizens, but also for the health and well-being of America's international image. Now, more than at any other time in the last several decades, is the time to show the world that Americans are willing to reach across borders and positively influence the welfare and health of all people, and in so doing, be good international citizens.

The passion of Rob's narrative touches all the concepts—intellectual, behavioral, and emotional—that have been formulated by the students' expectations in all the service-centered endeavors. The reaffirmation of the deeply felt desire to serve the vulnerable and disenfranchised, the invaluable aspect of being actively involved, the bonding that evolves from true collegiality, the citizen-of-the-world perspective instilled by volunteering in developing countries, the inspiration from the broadening of his personal perspective on life and career—all are integrated in an idealistic family doctor who epitomizes the core values of medicine that have been given so much attention recently. Moreover, Rob states unequivocally that RCSIP and RSIHM have been the vehicles that provided the opportunity to pursue those values that constitute the moral basis of being a physician (Eckenfels and Addington 1999). Rob had also been an Albert Schweitzer Fellow where he along with the other participants, embraced Schweitzer's "reverence for life."

Geeta has strong ties with her family in India. Prior to medical school, she had gone there and served as a health care worker in Haripuram, a small village one hundred miles from the nearest town. She eventually visited Cuba and worked there:

As medical school was coming to a close I was becoming increasingly aware that America's health care system, while advanced in its methods and medicines, was severely lacking in its ability to reach the masses. I had read an essay by the Institute of Social Justice on Cuba's low infant morality rate, exceptional control of the spread of HIV, and universal health care system. I was intrigued as to how all of this could exist in the face of U.S. economic sanctions that had been in place since the 1960s. I lived on campus at a Cuban medical school, went to classes on public health and the Cuban health care system, and worked alongside a Cuban doctor. What I found in Cuba was truly amazing. Here all medical students do a primary care residency before any other. The country was divided into four-block-by-four-block zones with each zone having a doctor that lived in a duplex above the clinic so your doctor was a member of your community. Any issue that concerned you as a citizen concerned you as a doctor as well. The elderly belonged to government-sponsored neighborhood social organizations that included daily exercise and outings. Pregnant women in need of extra care could live in a maternity home where a doctor would see them daily and they would be fed and taken care of. All day care centers were run by doctors and teachers, and children were taught that breastfeeding, self-care, and care of one's family were important and necessary parts of life. My experience here was unbelievable! Basically, I saw that the health needs of a society depended entirely on the government's dedication to universal access to care even despite scarce resources.

Cuban people have suffered tremendously under U.S. sanctions, but their infant mortality rate is far lower than that of the U.S. because the Cuban government places social justice in high regard. After being a part of that kind of system and seeing that even a poor country like Cuba was keeping its citizens healthy, I felt a new sense of commitment to the cause of universal care in America. It can work. And nothing can make you believe more than going to a place and seeing for yourself.

Geeta certainly puts her practice where her values are. As a family doctor with specialty training in maternal and child care, she delivers babies and looks after migrant workers in Southern California, where she lives with her husband, also a physician, and their two children. She also speaks openly and freely about her political action and its essential role in universal health care.

Did our service-learning programs radicalize Geeta? The fire was there, and with RCSIP she simply fanned the flames. Again, we see in these community service and health experiences the intertwining of one's personal beliefs with one's vocation. These two narrators' own words offer a glimpse of how their nascent idealism and compassion were cultivated through active participation in RCSIP and RSIHM.

Unfortunately, the good intentions to maintain, let alone expand, international health were thwarted by a number of unforeseen factors. Since the late 1990s payment for hospital services by major insurance providers—private and government—began dropping below the bottom line. Sustainability of the institution took precedence over everything else except patient care. Rush was only one of many hospitals facing this situation, and during the financial crunch many across the country were closed.

Although an Office of International Health was established at Rush (and was a natural home for RSIHM), its top priority became attracting financially solvent foreign patients to the medical center for advanced technical procedures. Under the pressure of a market-driven health care system, sponsoring a major new student program was given low priority. Without funding, RSIHM was not able to continue on its own. Furthermore, although I was designing a method to demonstrate the efficacy of RSIHM, it was fruitless to evaluate a program longitudinally that didn't even have the resources to sustain itself. Some of the highlights from the three years (1997–1999) during which RSIHM was fully functioning illustrate the worthiness of such programs.

As I put the brief history of RSIHM into perspective, a number of things become clear. It was apparent from the start that RSIHM was a costly undertaking. Although living accommodations in developing countries may be cheap by our standards, getting to and from those countries is not. As the faculty advisor to the group, my responsibility was to get formal recognition of the organization by the dean's office along with financial support. Dean Brueschke was very receptive to the idea of a student international health group but was limited with respect to the level of funding he could provide. He felt that the best and most equitable thing he could do was offer four fellowships for international health annually. Although we were very grateful to the dean, this raised a serious dilemma for the group. One of our fundamental aims was to get as many students as possible overseas, and if the only source of funding was summer fellowships awarded on merit, it meant that the students would be competing among themselves. The basic foundation of RSIHM, as for RCSIP, rests on cooperation rather than competition. Moreover, it was our contention that universal human rights, especially social justice, are sustained by teamwork, since a collaborative approach reinforces the courage needed to confront real humanitarian issues in health and welfare in poor and underdeveloped countries.

The students' solution to this dilemma was to divide all funds equally among those who demonstrated a serious commitment to work abroad over the summer. Since four fellowships ($2,500 each) would not be enough to send the ten to fifteen students overseas, it was further decided that the group had to engage in some fund-raising activities of its own and create a mechanism for an equitable distribution of the money. I found this an extremely admirable undertaking. It is an excellent example of participatory democracy in action. That is, the students were committed to working together to reach their goal. Below, I provide a summary of key achievements.

Our organizational accomplishments were as follows:

- We surveyed and listed forty-three faculty members with international health ties.
- We collected and organized brochures, reports, and a newsletter as well as pertinent information on the customs, laws, culture, values,

health conditions, visa requirements and the like to be maintained as an archive.

- A guidebook was created and placed in the university library for easy access.
- We established protocols for orientation, participation, and assessment; these are also kept in the library.
- A list of requirements was solicited, to ensure the safety of students going into developing countries, from International Health and Medical Education—the major organization for medical schools dedicated to international health activities.
- We recruited a faculty advisory committee of six individuals who had personal contacts in developing countries.
- Two student leaders were selected from the M1 and M2 classes who would have the responsibility of making RSIHM a student-generated, student-run, self-sustaining organization.
- We received recognition as a student organization by the dean.
- We initiated and engaged in fund-raising activities to supplement the summer fellowships.
- A mechanism for equitable distribution of funds was developed.

Experience outcomes were as follows:

- During this three-year period about fifty students went abroad, thirty of them between their M1 and M2 years.
- Twenty percent of the 1999 M1 class belonged to RSIHM.
- A series of fund-raising activities raised $3,000 (1997), $10,000 (1998), and $15,000 (1999).
- A journal club was established and met at least once a quarter to review evolving information on international health opportunities and barriers.
- Student-faculty luncheons, sponsored by my office, were started.
- A group of students presented a poster describing the development, operation, and goals of RSIHM at the 1999 annual International Health and Medical Education Conference in San Diego.
- The student participants spent a summer in many different countries, among them South Africa, Costa Rica, Mexico, Guatemala, Colombia, Haiti, Serbia, India, Korea, Vietnam, Indonesia, and China.

In conclusion, Rush medical students demonstrated their ability to establish a new approach to personal learning and development through immersion in another culture. RSIHM, in the spirit of volunteerism, provided students with international health experiences starting in their M1 year that remained independent of a formal elective with particular requirements. The initiative served as an educational innovation by promoting cultural awareness, altruism, humanism, and social responsibility. However, with the closing of the International Health Office there was no infrastructure for RSIHM to attach to. Since international health ventures are costly, some form of subsidy would have had to be found to revive the program. But as with RCSIP, the variety of international activities, the wealth of experiences, and the extent of commitment demonstrated the substance of what student-generated, voluntary health care services were able to achieve outside the confines of the traditional American medical education and delivery system.

One final note: The end of RSIHM didn't end students' search for international health experiences. Every year some students go abroad even on their own. The archives of information started by the original group is still maintained and updated. Faculty members still help students with placements and, in some instances, financial support. If the modern world is flat, to quote Thomas Friedman, then there will always be Rush students looking for horizons.

Chapter 6

Looking for Meaning

To reduce the totality of these experiences
to that mere portion of reality that is measurable is to deprive authentic development
of its fullness and to falsify reality itself.

—Dennis Goulet, "An Ethical Model for the
Study of Values"

Since RCSIP emerged spontaneously, evolving rapidly out of student enthusiasm, it was impossible to prepare any truly systematic evaluation scheme in
advance. Yet the questions that are most frequently asked are about evaluation—what kind of controls, if any, were used, what were the outcomes, what
measurements were used, what statistical methods were applied—that is, the
standard questions found in formal grant proposals that, by definition, impose
a specific protocol for program evaluation. Program efficacy is judged on measurable outcomes. The types and numbers of services rendered can be classified
and counted and thus are quantifiable. Participants' actions and behaviors are
measured by preconceived observational checklists, whereas attitudes, values,
and beliefs rely on responses acquired through questionnaires and, when feasible, interview schedules. While the interviews are considered qualitative, the
response rates can be quantified and subjected to statistical analysis. The proof is
in the p value. The results are used to make generalizations, frequently couched
in terms of causality. What makes this method untenable for my purposes is the

rigid belief in numbers as "scientific proof." If the program doesn't fit into a statistical format, it is considered anecdotal at best. (A cursory review of articles in medical education journals makes my point.) From my perspective, the same measurement hang-up has become the bane of designing, implementing, and assessing pedagogical innovations in medical education. Too often the method wags the program.

This methodology has major limitations when it comes to grasping the full essence of what RCSIP accomplished with respect to the learning and development of the student participants. The traditional research model described above insulates the evaluators from what they are trying to evaluate. The rich substance of meaning found in the complex series of events, interactions, and experiences for the RCSIP activists is best captured in narratives, face-to-face talks, keen observations, and purposeful thinking that are reflective and deductive. When I was approached by the students to help facilitate RCSIP, I accepted immediately because I knew, intuitively, à la Malcolm Gladwell's best-selling book *Blink* (2005), that it was a "good thing." It was in the process of program activity that I recognized its full significance in the students' maturation, as they moved toward becoming humane and compassionate doctors.

Before I continue, I need to say a few things about the narratives. First, for me, narratives have always been like what Paul Simon sings about, "windows to the heart": they express what is deeply felt by the narrator. Arthur Kleinman's *Illness Narratives* (1988), considered a hallmark work on patients' narratives, is a wonderful example of the power of narratives applied to health and illness. In an insightful essay, Rita Charon (1993) writes that narratives "all bear the stamp of their tellers, who are not detached observers, but who actively participate in generating the stories they tell" (149). Although Charon is focusing on the patient's "narrative road to empathy," her grasp, like Kleinman's, of the *substance* of the narrative demonstrates how valuable it is at getting at the emotional and cognitive basis of who the person is who is giving the self-narration. Narratives, outside their power in a novel or biography, have been discounted in much of social research in medical education because they do not fit the logicoscientific model. But as the cognitive psychologist Benedict Carey (2007) points out in a recent *New York Times* piece, "In the past decade or so a handful of psychologists have argued that the quicksilver elements of *personal narratives* belong in any three-dimensional picture of personality" (italics added). Researchers in psychology have found that the human brain has a natural affinity for narrative construction. In this regard, I have always found it disconcerting that researchers are willing to accept scores on attitude scales or precoded responses as representing the full meaning of what a respondent thinks or feels in great personal detail.

Therefore, this book is interspersed with narratives from students, faculty, patients or clients, and community representatives. These include some *unsolicited* comments that I recorded after the fact and those I purposefully *solicited* from active RCSIP participants. I am sure it is obvious that the faculty members were seasoned veterans who had a stake in RCSIP from the start, but who call it as they see it. The group that I concentrated on most were activists who are now practicing physicians. However, I had some difficulty getting responses to my e-mail requests: the alumni office didn't have current addresses and I couldn't find them on my own; some simply said they were overwhelmed at the moment and would write later but didn't; and there were some narratives that repeated what others had said, so I excluded them. Therefore, you can say my sample is a biased one, but nonetheless, the narratives tell the full story of the impact that RCSIP had on the respondents both personally and professionally. I could go on and on about their being in the early stages of their career, starting a family (a few mentioned that), ending up in graduate medical education programs that constrained their social action, and so on. These are realities that those of us who have been analyzing medical education know and must deal with on a routine basis. Regardless, the narratives speak for themselves and, hopefully, reinforce our own motivation to see them as a catalyst for reform. This is my main reason for writing this book.

While I am thinking along these lines, I also realize there is a certain repetitiveness when it comes to making points I want to reinforce, especially regarding fostering humanism and understanding cultural constructs and class differences. But the significance of how these values are cultivated subjectively in different situations and circumstances justifies this repetition.

The dual nature of RSCIP—service and learning—complicated the process of evaluation. First, it was necessary to distinguish between service and learning to show how they interacted and combined (see chart 1). Second, the quantitative aspect of assessment had to be integrated with the qualitative aspect. The former was based on those factors that could be measured (number of patients seen at a particular clinic) and those factors that could be compared (academic performance of different groups of student participants). The latter referred to unsolicited commentaries, open discussions, probed responses, personal narratives, and continual observations pertaining to the values, attitudes, and expectations that were elicited and catalogued by the program directors. In other words, these were not responses to an attitude scale or a series of precoded questions; they were full expressions of thoughts and feelings.

The purpose of the service component is to make available health care and advice to the underserved and marginalized. There are two ways in which this

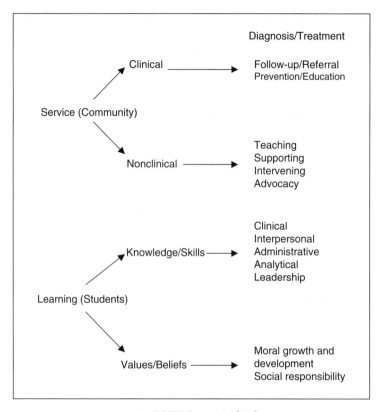

Chart 1 RCSIP Conceptual Schema

was accomplished. The first was through patient-oriented acts, which included treating the illness (whether chronic or acute), alleviating the pain and suffering (palliative care), preventing further illness (controlling disease), and providing comfort and reassurance (respect and empathy). The second was through programmatic acts, that is, teaching basic wellness skills (health promotion), developing interventions (safe sex), and initiating and supporting community activities (asthma camp). All these actions took place in the community, at clinics (neighborhood, public health), at community centers (Boys and Girls Clubs, homeless shelters), at homes (housing projects, family shelters), and anywhere the opportunity arose (health fairs, schools).

To appreciate the full extent of the clinical exposure of the students, it is important to reiterate that in the late 1980s and early 1990s placing students in ambulatory settings was considered interference in patient care, since it slowed down the physician, reduced the number of patients being seen, and detracted from the quality of care being delivered. It was further seen as an inconvenience to the patients and, in some quarters, was viewed as a form of guinea-pigging; that is, students were learning on the poor and most vulnerable patients (the St. Basil's attitude). Despite these concerns, there was, and still is, a desperate need to deliver medical services to large segments of the population (the homeless, recent immigrants, the uninsured) that are without any form of health care. The students sincerely believed and demonstrated that they, with the support and guidance of physician teachers and other concerned faculty, could help fill this gap. In some situations this took the form of actually starting a clinic project where none had existed before.

There is, however, one caveat to keep in mind. It is impossible to measure what impact these interventions are going to have in the long run. This is not to downplay the services being provided. One important aspect, indeed a major aim of the programs, is to expose future doctors to what it is like to be poor, a member of a minority group, and uninsured. In the process of helping those in need, humanistic values are fostered and idealism is nurtured.

By focusing primarily on the aggregate rather than on the individual, the nonclinical activities reflected a population and community perspective. Since the participants were medical students, they automatically related the nonclinical experiences to their role as future physicians. They saw the potential power of health education at the community level as a mechanism for disease prevention and wellness promotion. Moreover, they were exposed to the power of culture as a filter for better understanding resistance to change, which is deeply ingrained in traditional health beliefs and habits. Their AIDS prevention and safe-sex courses that were geared primarily toward inner-city kids is an excellent example in this regard. The tutoring programs gave the medical students insights into life in the housing projects and how social and economic factors such as no father at home and being on welfare related to physical and mental health. In short, they experienced health and illness from a social and cultural perspective.

Jackie Reed, a leading community organizer and the executive director of the West Side Health Authority, eloquently defined the meaning of health care from the community's perspective in 2002:

> Health care is not just a matter of going to the doctor. It should also be a source of healing for the community in general and empowering the disenfranchised. Many of the problems of health in this country, I think, are related to social ills in society—poor education, poor housing, poor job opportunities, and lack of community. What I mean by that is there is a lack of social networks and social relationships that make people feel better emotionally about themselves, about their neighborhoods,

about their circumstance, regardless of their socioeconomic condition. At the same time, the things that really produce health, such as stable communities, good education and job opportunities, good relationships, good park districts in a neighborhood, have consistently been neglected over the past fifty years in American society.

Reed is a strong advocate for creating partnerships between local communities and social institutions. RCSIP was seen as such a partner in her scheme of things. She promotes community empowerment "one block at a time."

Like the service component, the learning component consists of two parts: the acquisition of knowledge and skills and the nurturing of attitudes and beliefs. There are four specific sets of skills that the students learned through participation in RCSIP: clinical, in patient care settings; administrative, in the organization and operation of the various projects; interpersonal, in relating to colleagues, peers, and clients; and analytical, in understanding relationships between socioeconomic status and physical health.

The development of clinical skills was made evident in the medical service settings. Medical students were actually engaged in providing rudimentary health care during their first and second years of medical school. They worked as a team, they were closely supervised, and they were given an introduction to the fundamental steps that constitute clinical judgment. Furthermore, all the RCSIP members who participated in AIDS projects, especially those who served as a big sib to a kid who was HIV positive, became, through their own initiative, quite knowledgeable about the etiology of the disease.

Administrative skills were essentially developed on the job. The program designers had to organize, execute, and maintain a complex operation from scratch while they were full-time medical students—a tremendous undertaking!

Interpersonal skills were essential not only for the students' communicating among themselves but also for their relating to patients and clients. These skills were especially prominent with respect to leadership that emerged from one's ability to make things function and to explain the function to others (Kolb 1984). The leaders demonstrated their ability to master the task at hand and in addition explained to their peers in a nonthreatening way what needed to be done and how to do it. The experience of RCSIP offers strong evidence that effective behavior, problem solving, and task assignment rest on the ability to relate to others. RCSIP tapped the unbridled potential of these bright young men and women.

Analytical skills involved participants' ability to see the relationship between culture, social status, and health (Cohen 2004). Furthermore, these nonbiomedical factors came to be understood not merely as population variables in an epidemiological sense but as constituting a condition that affected the life and well-being of the community or social group members.

If my thesis is credible, then I want to reemphasize an important point: to be taken seriously as an exercise in learning through doing, RCSIP must be judged for its contribution to an understanding of how student participation cultivated, reinforced, and sustained the primary values and beliefs in which American medicine is so deeply invested. In addition, to prove its efficacy it must demonstrate that the attitudes and beliefs spawned through these experiences were fostered in social reality. In other words, the student participants were able to see and think outside the academic medicine box. Community service thus enabled them to become aware of the fact, too often ignored, that basic human needs—health and well-being—are not being met if you are at the bottom of the social stratification system (Marmot 2004).

The trickiest and most challenging area for conceptualization lies in how to determine the conditions that have fostered humanistic values, attitudes, and beliefs. For starters, it seemed apparent that for students to want to initiate a community service program, some attributes, such as compassion and caring, were already there. Volunteerism is laden with emotion: it comes from the heart. In this context I saw volunteerism as giving the medical students an opportunity to express their idealism personally and collectively. By giving of themselves freely outside the formal educational system, the participants attested to what Robert Coles (1993) has observed: "Service is a means of putting to use what we have learned—to connect moral ideals to the lived life."

Development is, above all, a question of values (Goulet 1971). One of the problems with the study of values is that they are considered to be best understood in rational or concrete terms. It is assumed that without such a framework, it would be impossible to determine what they are. When values are perceived as tangible, rational entities, it is also assumed that they can be taught like any other body of knowledge. This is a mistake made too often in medical education. A course in medical ethics clearly does not make one ethical. The Association of American Medical Colleges (Medical School Objectives Project [MSOP] 1998) and other professional bodies subscribe to the notion that values, among them altruism and dutifulness, can be taught like any other didactic topic. If values are learned this way, they become static and factual.[1]

In actuality, values evoke feelings that Martha Nussbaum (2001) calls "emotional intelligence." "Emotions," she believes, "involve judgments of important things" (19). They alert us to what matters most. Nussbaum gives special attention to compassion and its role in public life. Her conceptualization, wonderfully stated in the title of her book, *Upheavals of Thought,* has particular merit for explaining how RCSIP participants put into action what they felt. The very nature of RCSIP's brand of voluntary community service represents an act of compassion in public life, whereas teaching medical ethics or professionalism in a didactic format keeps the subject detached from its emotional underpinnings.

Since altruism is considered one of the four objectives of becoming a truly competent physician (MSOP 1998), Nussbaum's observations on compassion and altruism are particularly relevant. She notes that compassion as translated into a beneficent act involves three judgments: (1) the seriousness of the misfortune of others is evident, (2) the misfortunes were not brought on by the victims themselves, and (3) alleviating the misfortunes is an important part of one's own scheme of ends and goals. She goes on to state, "The conjunction of these beliefs is very likely to lead to action addressing the suffering" (335). In RCSIP, the students feel compassionate and act altruistically.

Nussbaum also raises the possibility that compassion, and the feelings it nourishes, can be a kind of self-interested reasoning. (This is the question Tracy Kidder raises to Paul Farmer, as discussed in the introduction.) This is an important point. To address it, I have looked deep into my own motivations and why I continued to engage in social action via community service when there is frequently no discernible impact of my efforts in terms of actually changing the wider system as it exists. What does become clear, however, is that regardless of the degree of immediate impact, I share a great feeling of satisfaction from giving myself openly in an attempt to help others. These experiences fit Nussbaum's observation that "the compassionate person is keenly aware of the distinction between her own life and that of the sufferer" (336). The ambivalence about our effectiveness (as change agent or Good Samaritan) is a great source of contemplation and reflection. These emotions are something other than rational judgments; they are a kind of pain caused by witnessing the plight of others.

RCSIP is also an excellent example of how empathy for the patient or client without access to needed resources typically leads to compassion and altruism and hence to helping the whole person. To use Nussbaum's notion, "people who attend to the distress of another in a manner sufficient for compassion have motives to help that person" (336). I contend that RCSIP participation tended to broaden, reinforce, and stabilize elements of concern that were already there. It is the idealism that was enhanced. Moreover, continued participation has the potential of creating a lasting ethical concern for others. What is important for this analysis, and at the center of my argument, is that RCSIP provided opportunities that facilitated altruistic and compassionate motives on the part of the student participants. In essence, it facilitated moral growth and intellectual development, the missing ingredients that the return to profession-alism is based on.

RCSIP involvement also built a strong sense of social responsibility that is fundamental to a democratic society in which political, social, and economic institutions are interconnected for a common good. This theme is woven throughout the students'—now doctors'—narratives. Since the concept of med-icine as a public trust (Schroeder, Zones, and Showstack 1989) until quite recently had not been examined critically but tended to be taken for granted and was showing clear signs of erosion, it is a worthwhile contribution to expose students to this responsibility early in their education. In this regard, I felt that it was important to put more emphasis on the social responsibility of the health professional in the community setting than on the doctor-patient relationship. This is in keeping with the great medical educator Lowell T. Coggeshall's concept of the physician as "an agent of society, licensed by society, to serve society before serving himself" (Howell 1992, 714). In helping students frame the unique features of RCSIP, I focused on being accountable to society, because the doctor-patient relationship is already inherent in the for-mal training of the physician; that is, it is the context in which one acquires clinical competence independent of social and other strictly nonmedical considerations. Although there is justifiable concern that in the training of the modern physician too much weight is put on the procedure and too little on the patient, limited attention is given to being responsible for the health of the whole society.

It is most enlightening to recognize the wonderful fluidity of the programs. RCSIP's strength—its persistence, purpose, and continuity—rested with the students' sense of ownership. The services offered to individual patients in clinic settings or groups in community-oriented endeavors continued to evolve of their own volition. Four fundamental skills of a competent health profes-sional for the twenty-first century—clinical, administrative, interpersonal, and analytical—were sharpened in the process. In the realm of developing core val-ues, RCSIP served as a mechanism for putting one's feelings into action. Claudia and I knew what was going on but were frustrated by the need to find some way of demonstrating what we saw as participant-observers.

I presume one could argue that I put the evaluation section after the fact. But after much consideration and consultation, I decided that the evaluation issue made more sense, that is, is more relevant, following a description of the programs as a whole. Therefore, in addressing the evaluation question even after the fact I delineated five distinct cohorts: (1) the patients and clients, in terms of actual numbers receiving care or education, their health status, and any outcomes that resulted from the care or education they received; (2) the students, with respect to their academic performance in medical school, their career choices, and their attitudes and beliefs; (3) the faculty, with respect to their personal satisfaction and role identity (mentor) as program participants; (4) the community, through its own representatives, as demonstrated by their support of the program; and (5) the program directors, from their special vantage point of seeing the program evolving from the start. Cohorts 1 and 2 are dealt with in the following two chapters. The observations of the faculty, community representatives, and the program directors are intertwined throughout the book.

Chapter 7

Empirical Estimates of Patients and Clients Served

Medicine has indeed delivered effective answers to some health problems and it has found the means to lessen the symptoms of many others, but by and large we remain with the necessity to do something about the incidence of disease, and that means a new partnership between health-services and all those whose decisions influence the determinants of its incidence.

—Geoffrey Rose, *The Strategy of Preventive Medicine*

The task of accounting for those people served by RCSIP is an interesting one. First, on the basis of my decision to limit and discuss in detail four very different and particularly revealing types of programs, I excluded a number of other activities that were just as important to the participants and the people they served. Second, for this assessment I have included all twenty-four programs that had been undertaken during the decade of the 1990s (see table 1). Third, there was no way to keep track of every individual seen in the twenty-four projects that ran between three and ten years of the decade of analysis. Fourth, at that time RCSIP had neither the personnel nor the funds to keep such records, let alone analyze them. Nonetheless, it is possible to offer estimates based on the evidence we have.

Table 1   **Rush Community Service Initiatives Program Projects, 1990–2000**

Project	Title	Purpose
AIDS	RAIDS	Teaching safe sex and AIDS prevention in inner-city schools
	Big Sib	Befriending HIV-positive infants and children in institutional care
	The AIDS Prevention Magic Show	Teaching AIDS prevention to youngsters
Clinic	St. Basil's Free People's Clinic	Developing a general medicine clinic in the Englewood community
	St. Basil's Free People's Clinic	Establishing a prenatal and gynecology clinic in the same community
	CommunityHealth	Providing primary care to a large Latino population
	Franciscan Homeless Clinic	Providing acute and primary care to the homeless
	Pilsen Homeless Shelter	Delivering primary and acute care to the homeless
Health education	Henry Horner Pediatric Asthma Program	Training local residents to serve as case managers and advocates for asthmatic children
	Rush Health Educators	Initiating health promotion training in schools
	Deborah's and Mariah's Place	Providing health education and support for abused and homeless women
Tutoring and mentoring	Henry Horner Tutoring	Tutoring and counseling children after school
	Buddies	Developing personal friendships with chronically ill children
	Casa Juan Diego	Tutoring Mexican children in the Pilsen community
Special	Refugee Young Gang Prevention	Working with refugees in Bosnian, Guatemalan, and Haitian communities
	Horizon Camp	Becoming involved with disabled children at summer camp
	Youth Link	Promoting patient education for adolescents at Stroger Hospital
	Casa Guatemala	Conducting screening and health evaluations with recent immigrants
	Frazier Elementary School Health Clinic	Providing health education and disease prevention by an interdisciplinary team

(Continued)

Table 1   (Continued)

Project	Title	Purpose
	ASAP	Teaching hospitalized adolescents about substance abuse and following their progress
	Mammovan	Participating in a mammogram van that reaches young women and girls on the West Side
	IHPP	Developing an interdisciplinary team from all of the university's colleges to provide health care to the poor and disadvantaged
	One Shot Deals	Conducting health fairs, school physicals, and immunizations
	Functional assessment of the elderly	Creating a checklist of daily activities as a way of assessing the needs of elderly patients

RCSIP served four general medicine clinics where patients were seen at least one day a week for eight years: St. Basil's, CommunityHealth, Franciscan, and Pilsen. The only realistic way of estimating the number of patient contacts is to establish ranges as a basis for calculating averages. The following formula was used in making estimates for each clinical setting: the range of the number of patients seen in one day times the number of days in an average year of operation times the number of years the project had been in operation. The mean number of contacts is reached by dividing the range by two. Applying the formula to the Rush General Medicine Clinic at St. Basil's serves as an example: between 8 and 15 patients were seen on one clinic day over an average of 42 days per year for 8 years; this number is then divided by two to determine the mean:

$$(8–15) \times 42 = (336–630) \times 8 = (2{,}688–5{,}040) \div 2 = 3{,}864$$

Using the same formula, with slight variations in numbers of patients seen and clinic days per year, we arrived at the following averages and ranges: CommunityHealth 5,000 (4,000–6,000), Pilsen 3,456 (3,072–3,840), and Franciscan 3,240 (2,880–3,600). On the basis of these very conservative estimates, the average and total range of patient contacts for the four clinics over eight years is calculated at 15,560 (12,640–18,480). The actual number of patient contacts was probably much higher, but these estimates were extrapolated from the best data available.

Other settings in which patients were seen included One Shot Deals, functional assessment of the elderly, Casa Guatemala, and the prenatal clinic at St. Basil's. In the One Shot Deals program, teams of RCSIP students and physicians responded to the need to immunize kids prior to the start of the school year; they also worked at health fairs sponsored by churches and other civic organizations. We estimate that 1,250 (1,000–1,500) kids were immunized by RCSIP teams. Another 1,500 (1,000–2,000) people, mostly adults, were screened at the health fairs, which have been conducted since the program started in 1990. Again, we feel that both these estimates are quite conservative. The functional-assessment-of-the-elderly project ran for about two and a half years and involved about 750 patient contacts. At Casa Guatemala around 200 patients were screened over a three-day weekend for the purpose of getting baseline health data to use in obtaining some form of health care through existing public health agencies. The prenatal clinic at St. Basil's had at least 300 patient contacts during its three years of operation; 65 healthy babies were delivered at Rush with an average of about five visits per pregnant woman either at the clinic or at Rush. In total these projects account for an additional 4,025 (3,275–4,775) contacts. Based on these calculations, the total average is approximately 19,585 (15,915–23,255) patient contacts over a little more than ten years (see table 2).

It was impossible, however, to determine how many of these contacts were follow-ups. For those screened at health fairs the answer is none. For the pregnant women seen at St. Basil's the answer is all of them. In other words, they averaged about five visits per patient. The follow-up is high among those elderly patients who were seen at the Erie Health Center. The initial assessment of functional ability required another visit to determine how each patient was doing. On average the same patients were seen by the student assessors at least twice.

Based on our observation and the estimates of the physician participants and the students, about half the patients seen at the four general medicine clinics were women, a third were children, and the rest were men. There was a follow-up to the initial encounter for between a quarter and a third of the patients. The three most common ailments for adults were, in rank order, hypertension, diabetes, and upper respiratory infections. Besides well-child visits, upper respiratory infections and digestive tract problems were the primary causes that brought children to the clinic. Parasites were also common, as were skin infections. This does not mean to suggest that all patient assessments were routine. There were some very sick people who required hospitalization or further extensive evaluation by specialists with access to advanced technology.

Table 2   **Estimates of Patient Contacts Seen by RCSIP Participants,**
1990–2000

Clinic	PT Range	Days	Years	Average (Range)
St. Basil's	8–15	42	8	3,864 (2,688–5,040)
ComH	10–15	50	8	5,000 (4,000–6,000)
Pilsen	8–10	48	8	3,456 (3,072–3,840)
Fran	8–10	45	8	3,240 (2,880–3,600)
			Subtotal 15,560 (12,640–18,480)	

Program	PT Range
Immuniz	1,250 (1,000–1,500)
One Shot	1,500 (1,000–2,000)
Func assess	750
Ob/gyn	325
Casa Guat	200
Subtotal 4,025 (3,275–4,775)	
GRAND TOTAL 19,585 (15,915–23,255)	

Note

St. Basil's= St. Basil's Free People's Clinic; ComH = CommunityHealth; Pilsen = Pilsen Homeless Shelter; Fran = Franciscan Homeless Shelter; Immuniz = Immunizations of children prior to starting school; One Shot = One Shot Deals; Func assess = Functional assessment of elderly patients; Ob/gyn = Ob/gyn clinic at St. Basil's; Casa Guat = Casa Guatemala.

The ethnicity of clinic patients was fairly evenly divided between Latinos (mostly of Mexican origin but quite a few from Central America) and African Americans. Many of the Latino patients were recent immigrants and had difficulty with English, but this situation increased the students' incentive to learn Spanish, especially medical Spanish. The condition common to them all was abject poverty or subsistence living at best and lack of access to health care. Obesity was commonplace, and smoking was prevalent among men (see table 3).

The medical services delivered were largely acute care management, school physicals, and immunizations. Since we emphasized disease prevention and heath promotion, RCSIP participants gave some attention to trying to get people to quit smoking, lose weight, and make some changes in their style of living. To help in this regard, RCSIP participants provided nutritional counseling, emphasized the importance of exercise, and offered acknowledged useful techniques for stress reduction. Health education in the form of counseling was also offered around such topics as reproductive health, the symptoms of asthma, sickle-cell anemia, and other health conditions that are common among poor minority people with limited education but are rarely diagnosed

Table 3   Demographic Profile of Clinic Patient Contacts, 1990–2000

Fairly evenly divided between African Americans and Latinos (the majority from Mexico or Central America with some undocumented immigrants)

35% children; 50% women; 15% men

Living conditions resulting from limited education and job skills

Majority uninsured working poor

Obesity widespread among children as well as adults

Less than half of the patients kept follow-up visits

Major ailments: hypertension, diabetes, upper respiratory[a]

Health education: anatomy, asthma, sickle cell anemia, family planning, communication skills

Disease prevention and health promotion: diet, exercise, smoking cessation, safe sex

Note

This profile does not include patients screened at health fairs or other mass screenings.

[a] Patients with serious heart conditions, neurological problems, and gastrointestinal illness were also seen.

by the overworked health care providers who treat them. The students quickly learned the limitations of offering health care in an environment in which living conditions play such an important role in the state of health and well-being. This was not a source of discouragement but instead a realistic assessment. Intervention for health and wellness is not simply providing medications and giving advice.

The majority of the sixty-five pregnant women seen at St. Basil's were Latinos, single, and young and experiencing their first pregnancy. The elderly patients seen at the Erie clinic were in their seventies and eighties, but a few were in their nineties. While most of them lived in senior housing, a number still lived with their extended families.

The essence of these contacts cannot be understood solely in medical and demographic terms, since the students spent a lot of time talking with the patients. What the students experienced, what they absorbed, was an understanding not only of the structure of poverty, but also of the hopes and aspirations of people who had limited access to opportunities for education and employment.

The nonmedical activities that RCSIP participants engaged in had tremendous value in their own right for future doctors. Students worked as hard at teaching, supporting, advising, and counseling and with as much vigor and compassion as they did administering medical services. The RAIDS teams reached about 1,750 (1,500–2,000) kids with their message. The magic show reached another 400 (300–500). Between 75 and 100 kids with AIDS were matched with a medical student big sib.

Safe sex and AIDS prevention were also included in the health promotion and education that was established at Crane and Frazier schools. (These relatively new programs grew out of earlier work in the school system.) Moreover, the health education provided by this group of RCSIP volunteers was open and straightforward. As described in chapter 3, when discussing human sexuality, they frequently used models to teach anatomy, and, when appropriate, they showed how to use a condom and other forms of birth control. When talking about what smoking or alcohol can do to the human body, they used actual diseased human organs. Since the medical students were young and energetic, they were able to create a lasting rapport with the children. They learned to talk the talk with the toughest of them.

RCSIP participants discussed asthma, substance abuse, and sexually transmitted diseases with children and, in some cases, their parents or guardians. The Buddies program followed chronically ill children in the same way the Big Sib project helped young victims of AIDS. Rush students worked with disabled youngsters at the Horizon camp, and RCSIP participants have also served as counselors at the asthma camp for Horner children.

But it is not only children who were served. At Deborah's Place and Mariah's Place, two shelters with permanent housing for homeless and abused women, RCSIP participants gave counseling and support. With Bosnian refugees the Rush team found resources to help parents and their children suffering from posttraumatic stress disease. The RCSIP participants learned that the Guatemalans they saw, most of Mayan descent, were victims of an oppressive government who had sought political asylum in churches on the Northwest Side. The students had firsthand exposure to their strength and their fortitude—an experience they will always remember. The control of asthma in the Henry Horner projects was the result of getting the message out to the entire community through picnics, variety shows, special holiday events, and other social functions. Again, it is impossible to estimate how many people "got the message," but it was certainly in the hundreds. It is impossible to demonstrate that the message took, but the word was out and asthma was being talked about.

Furthermore, the tutoring projects initiated by RCSIP were highly successful in creating an atmosphere of warmth and affection. Some of the kids showed their report cards to the tutors if there was an improvement in their grades. Sitting down with a child or a small group and going over math problems or reading aloud to show the excitement of reading was a strong mechanism for bonding. Keep in mind that the medical students' success at tutoring

Table 4 **Estimates of Client Contacts by RCSIP Participants, 1990–2000**

RCSIP Project	Average (range) of Clients Seen
RAIDS	1,750 (1,500–2,000)
AIDS Big Sib	88 (75–100)
AIDS Magic	400 (300–500)
Childhood Asthma	125 (100–150)
Health Educators	500 (400–600)
Homeless and Abused Women	125 (100–150)
Horner Tutoring	400 (300–500)
Casa Juan Diego Tutoring	150 (125–175)
Buddies	75 (50–100)
Frazier School Clinic	125 (100–150)
TOTAL RANGE	3,738 (3,050–4,425)

Note

Clients tend to be poor, underrepresented minority children with the exception of young women found in homeless and abused-women's shelters.

in Henry Horner was the linchpin of creating the asthma program. The Rush students who currently tutor at Casa Juan Diego, a youth center sponsored by St. Pius Catholic Church in Pilsen, get the additional payoff of using their Spanish. This reciprocity is a great source of bonding as well. Based on estimates of these activities, I feel confident in saying that hundreds of people, mostly children, were reached through RCSIP's efforts at health promotion, counseling, support, tutoring, and mentoring (see table 4). Although these activities are not specifically medical, they at the core of giving care.

It is important to acknowledge that it is impossible to measure what impact these interventions are going to have in the long run. This is not to downplay the services that have been provided. These personal encounters exposed future doctors to what life is like outside the walls of the academic medical center. But the most fulfilling aspect of these activities, which is the focus of this book, is to see these kids laugh, carry on, and come up with the right answer, a wonderful reward in its own right. This process of helping those in need is a humanistic act in which idealism is nurtured.

Chapter 8

The Learning and Development of the Students

From early on, many medical students speak of a kind of "passion" required for doctoring. Not only do they seek a specialty that will maintain their intellectual excitement, but many describe their desire for a passionate engagement with the primal forces of sickness and suffering, a passionate struggle on behalf of their patients.

—Byron J. Good, *Medicine, Rationality, and Experience*

Academic Performance and Career Choice

When the fifth class with RCSIP representation graduated in 1994, it was possible to try to measure what, if any, effect participation was having on the students' academic performance. The total number of students who graduated in the five-year period 1990–1994 was 565, of which 176 (31 percent) participated at some level in RCSIP, despite RCSIP being still in its first stage of growth. The real participation explosion began in the second half of the 1990s. Furthermore, because the main thrust of this book is on the genesis of RCSIP, I felt I needed to tell the story of the early phase before its significance faded. Extrapolating meaning from human engagements in personal and social action requires considerable time and effort. The academic performance side of analysis, however, fits nicely into a quantitative format.

The five classes provided a clear distinction in degrees of participation. It was possible to divide the students into mutually exclusive groups: nonparticipants, those with no involvement in RCSIP, and participants, a group that was further divided into regular participants and activists. Members of the activist group were distinguished by a combination of factors—their role in initiating new programs, extent and duration of participation, membership in one of the RCSIP committees, formal presentations or published papers, and confirmation of their status by a survey of peers. The verification of these observations provided a high degree of reliability, making it possible to use the three categories as a correlation coefficient in our analysis. Our hypothesis was twofold: the greater the extent of participation in RCSIP, the better the students would perform overall academically and the more likely they would choose a primary care residency.

The format of analysis consisted of five components: (1) extent of participation, (2) grade-point averages (GPAs) and Medical College Aptitude Test (MCAT) scores, (3) course grades and United States Medical Licensing Examination (USMLE) scores, (4) dean's letter ratings, and (5) residency choice. In other words, the three groups were compared by standard performance measurements at matriculation to serve as baseline; course grades, certification scores, and class ranking served as an indication of academic performance throughout medical school; and residency selection was an indication of career choice. Preliminary statistical analysis showed that the level of program participation was partially related to gender and enrollment in the parallel track, the two-year, preclinical, problem-based learning program called the alternative curriculum. For this reason, all comparisons were conducted by means of an analysis of covariance in which gender (52 percent male, 48 percent female) and enrollment in the traditional curriculum or alternative curriculum (87 percent and 13 percent, respectively) served as covariants. Outcome data were adjusted for the effects of the covariants. The results of the analysis are summarized in table 5.

The small differences in total and science GPAs for all groups were not significant. A slight difference was found for MCAT scores. A gradient emerged in which the nonparticipants registered the highest scores and activists the lowest. The differences were statistically significant for chemistry and for problem solving and bordered on significant for biological and physical sciences. Taken together, however, these measures of academic achievement prior to medical school showed little to no difference among the three groups but slightly better scores for the nonparticipants in the science part of the MCAT. A separate analysis showed that there was no significant difference in undergraduate major or graduate degree. A comparison of academic performance scores in

Table 5   **Academic Performance Measures for Three Levels of RCSIP Participation**

	Nonparticipants (N = 389)	Participants (N = 120)	Activists (N = 56)	p-value
Prior to medical school				
Undergraduate GPA (science)	3.26	3.18	3.25	0.94
Undergraduate GPA (total)	3.33	3.28	3.37	0.136
MCAT				
Biological sciences	9.72	9.44	9.27	0.063
Chemistry	9.22	9.09	8.55	0.019
Physical sciences	9.21	8.93	8.75	0.064
Problem solving	9.17	8.95	8.61	0.024
Reading	8.43	8.32	8.56	0.733
Quantitative	8.29	8.22	8.06	0.683
During medical school				
Preclinical grades	2.31	2.3	2.48	0.086
USMLE, Step 1	196.4	202.1	199.2	0.009
Clinical grades	2.70	2.96	3.12	<.0001
Internal medicine	2.61	2.89	3.05	<.0001
Surgery	2.74	2.95	2.95	0.062
Pediatrics	2.6	2.84	2.99	<.0001
Family medicine	2.88	2.99	3.21	0.015
OB/Gyn	2.80	3.07	3.17	<.0001
Psychiatry	2.85	2.89	3.12	0.057
Neurology	3.00	3.23	3.30	<.0001
USMLE, Step 2	194.1	201.6	201.4	<.0001
Class rank (dean's letter)	67.7	52.81	44.65	<.0001
Primary care Specialty	37.80%	56.80%	73.20%	0.016

Note

Means adjusted by analysis of covariance for effects of gender and participation in problem-solving curriculum. Data include members of five sequential medical school classes (1990 to 1994).

medical school showed that activists had slightly higher preclinical grades, but the trend was not statistically significant. Both participants and activists achieved significantly higher scores on USMLE Step 1 than those of nonparticipants, but there was no real trend. In sum, there was little difference among the three groups at baseline and in preclinical academic performance.

In the clinical years, however, significant differences in academic performance did emerge. These trends were found in both composite and individual clerkship grades, which were higher for participants and activists as compared with nonparticipants, with the activists having the highest scores. This trend held for all seven core clerkships although not rising to the level of statistical significance for surgery and psychiatry. It seems reasonable to assume that surgery would not be high in the attainment of students interested in community health and ambulatory care. Lack of a significant difference in psychiatry was more perplexing. One possibility is that contemporary psychiatry relies more on psychopharmacology than on talk therapy, which could be an indication of why activists were not noticeably drawn to it. RCSIP participants did especially well in the primary care disciplines. USMLE Step 2 (clinical) scores follow the same pattern: both groups of participants scored higher than nonparticipants did.

The entire academic performance of a Rush medical student is summarized in the dean's letter. Rush, like most other medical schools, does not rank students numerically, but it does use course grades as a method for determining overall academic performance. (The total scores are converted to a percentile system in which the lower the percentile, the higher the standing in the class.) As a summary index, the dean's letter confirms the same pattern of academic performance by showing a clear linear relationship: activists received the highest ranking and the nonparticipants the lowest.

Of particular importance to Rush, because of its goal in the 1990s of having 50 percent of its graduates become generalists, is the choice of residencies. More than seven out of ten (73.2 percent) of the activists and more than half the participants (56.8 percent) as compared with one-third (38 percent) of the nonparticipants selected a primary care residency ($p = .016$).

The results of this evaluation showed that, despite no discernible difference in GPA and MCAT score among all three groups and controlling for gender and placement in the problem-based learning curriculum, there was a statistically significant difference between extent of participation in RCSIP and clinical clerkship grades and dean's letter rankings for the five classes. In addition, the same kind of relationship was found when extent of participation was applied to the graduates' selection of primary care residencies. In short, the greater the extent of participation in RCSIP, the higher the academic performance in the clinical rotations and the greater the likelihood of selecting a primary care residency.

It is impossible to prove that RCSIP participation resulted in good clinical grades and the selection of primary care residencies in any causal sense. Our findings, however, show one certainty: RCSIP participation did not detract from the students' academic performance despite the administration's initial concern. A reasonable explanation for the findings can be found through exclusion and deduction. Is it strictly by chance that RCSIP participants performed well on their clinical clerkships? And why was the percentage of participants and activists choosing primary care residencies so high?

There are clear factors for explaining the good clerkship performance. By working closely with their physician mentors in RCSIP-sponsored clinical projects, the students learned fundamental clinical skills that gave them an advantage over their nonparticipant peers in the clinical rotations. But it was more than the skills acquired taking physicals and histories. The students had already become comfortable in relating to patients and their families. Their confidence grew with each encounter with the patients, doctors, and the community. Before their first clerkship, many of them had already learned how to present themselves to patients in a manner that was sincere, culturally sensitive, and empathic, and they had done so in an atmosphere that was conducive to professional growth. Rush physicians who volunteered treated the students as junior colleagues.

In terms of residency choices, almost all the physicians who volunteered were generalists, mostly family practitioners, internists, and pediatricians. They were ideal mentors and role models for the students. They made primary care come alive. When the RCSIP clinical activities first began, the students were given an opportunity to engage patients on a personal level and discuss each case with one or more of their physician mentors. In other words, the students were afforded the time to learn how to practice medicine through personal contact with the patient and their mentor. This was in contrast to the impersonal medicine they saw in the academic health center.

Social Medicine and Community Health

Since these experiences took place at clinical sites located in disadvantaged neighborhoods, they also served as an apprenticeship for community health. The students saw their physician colleagues serving the community as well as the patient. Social responsibility was also an intrinsic lesson learned. They discovered that this was not only compassionate medicine but intellectually challenging medicine as well, because the patient's illness needed to be understood holistically. When it came to choosing graduate medical education programs, primary care became a logical extension of the students' community service efforts. Most of the activists looked for programs with a strong emphasis on ambulatory care in community clinics. In those clinics that were hospital based, they sought settings where they could use their awareness of the patients' cultural and social circumstances as a prerequisite for providing quality health care.

In the primarily social service activities and other nonclinical projects, the sense of purpose for becoming a physician was also reinforced. There the role of the physician as team leader was present. By being active in community settings, the students obtained firsthand exposure to what is needed and what can be done. In addition, they were able to feel welcome in such settings. Their actions resulted in being accepted by community residents, who saw them as advocates and partners working on their behalf. These relationships fostered a strong sense of commitment on the part of the students. They had a deep-seated motivation to work harder academically to become better doctors. The students were also seen by community leaders as ambassadors for the medical center; it was the Rush students who were there to help. This gave the students a sense of pride and identity. They loved to be referred to as "the Rush students."

All these activities took place in a supportive and collaborative atmosphere. The students were not competing among themselves; they were working together. They brought a sense of self-confidence, good interpersonal skills, and a cooperative attitude to the floors of the academic health center. These attitudes and their accompanying behaviors were demonstrated in their clerkship performance and recognized by their clerkship directors as clear signs of clinical competence.

The Subjective Factor

It is important to look behind the numbers to find out what these experiences really meant to the participants personally. In a dynamic and evolving social action program such as RCSIP, it is impossible to stop the process, take a slice of reality, and measure it in some quantitative manner. Even a well-designed questionnaire would have major limitations. The explanation lies in the process of participation. It is, nonetheless, impossible to differentiate between the reaffirmation of the students' values and aspirations and the initiation of new attitudes and beliefs. But in either case it was a developmental experience. For example, RCSIP gave some students, especially the original leaders, a chance to test their values and put them into action. For others, RCSIP exposed them to a totally new set of experiences outside their traditional ways of viewing the world and themselves. The students had to create an acceptable, effective, and sustainable program and recruit voluntary faculty to supervise them. In short, RCSIP required a major commitment on the part of the student participants, which had a powerful influence on them personally and professionally.

Trying to explain this phenomenon has important implications in its own right. I alluded to this in chapter 7. First, there is an obsession among many medical educators that quantification is the only way to determine if a relationship is valid. Program evaluators want it both ways: they want proof that A causes B, and, at the same time, they want to disprove any relationship that can't be considered causal. Even as we move toward ever finer calibrations of statistical measurement, the logicodeductive knowledge that social science can produce is, in the end, limited. By following these rigid, positivistic rules, the potential of such innovations as RCSIP would be discounted. In other words, there is no way of "objectively" proving their effectiveness in functional terms. The irony of this spurious-correlation kind of reasoning is that it is still maintained at a time when a major concern in medicine is the acquisition and affirmation of core values that constitute professionalism: the very kind of thing that does not fit such an analytical paradigm.

When it comes to assessing moral values and attitudes, we have to rely on other methods that are much more akin to what Ortner (2006) calls an "anthropology of subjectivity, both as states of mind of real actors embedded in the social world and as formulations that (at least partially) express, shape, and constitute those states of mind" (127). Goulet (1971) reminds us that "values belong to the realm of synthesis, not analysis. To reduce this synthesis to an instrumentality of arbitrary 'scientific rules' is to lose its fundamental symbolic meaning" (38).

The reference here is to a more analogical kind of thinking, that is, one for which metaphors, models, and narration provide the basis for understanding phenomena that do not adequately fit quantification. Physician anthropologists such as Kleinman (1995) and Farmer (2003) are well acquainted with the dominant biomedical paradigm and are especially astute at this interpretative approach. Following their lead, I aimed in my analysis for consistency, that is, the verification of the conceptual categories that organized my observations. This is important because the essence of my explanation is based on the participants' own interpretation of their experiences (their narratives) and how these affected their attitudes and behavior as future physicians and socially responsible citizens. My next task is to integrate these elements into a composite frame for understanding the growth and development of the student idealist as a catalyst for humanistic reform in medical education.

Chapter 9

Nurturing Idealism, Advancing Humanism, and Planning Reform

The organizational culture of medicine used to be dominated by the ideals of professionalism and voluntarism, which softened the underlying acquisitive activity. The restraint exercised by these ideals now grows weaker. The "health center" of one era is the "profit center" of the next.

—Paul Starr, *The Social Transformation of American Medicine*

The Elements That Matter

It is time to put what I have said so far into some kind of overarching framework. The four pillars of RCSIP—student initiated, student run, voluntary, and extracurricular—are the sine qua non of the program. An analysis of what constitutes RCSIP during its first decade must necessarily be concerned with an equation embracing at least four major elements: service, learning, values, and community. The biomedical side of the equation is already an established fixture in the formal medical school curriculum.

RCSIP students and faculty provided health care to thousands of poor members of ethnic minority groups living in disadvantaged communities and taught, counseled, and befriended thousands of kids. This constitutes the *service* side of the total equation. The communities where the broad range of programs took place welcomed the students openly and appreciated and fully used the service students offered. In some situations, RCSIP participants and the populations and communities they assisted developed partnerships and lasting bonds. The faculty mentors, like their student charges, remained deeply committed to their work. The program directors accepted the duty of guiding the program's functions and documenting its achievements.

Initially, my primary focus on the *learning* side was the benevolent nature of RCSIP's services as a means of fostering humanistic attitudes, and I neglected to give proper attention to the complex organizational structure that they had to create from scratch. The students had to work hard in designing and implementing specific duties and assignments to make RCSIP operational. Moreover, they had to create an atmosphere of trust among themselves, with the faculty they brought with them, and in the communities they served. They needed to share common goals and the means to achieve them. In the process of pursuing these goals, they were able to develop sound administrative and interpersonal skills, fostered through open communication. This spirit of cooperation bound them together on a deeply personal level. Recognized student leaders emerged in this process. As revealed in our study of academic performance, almost all of them displayed good to excellent clinical competence. Besides being enthusiastic about working as a team, being interpersonally connected, and giving service to the underserved, they lost their inhibitions about expressing their feelings, doubts, and ideals among those, particularly the program directors, who shared the same sentiments. They learned far more than I expected.

The *values* side of the equation required that I examine, as systematically as possible, the ideals that motivated the participants initially and subsequently. For a "total immersion" approach to a commitment to serve the poor, I turn again to Paul Farmer.[1] He has created community-based treatment strategies for tuberculosis, sexually transmitted infections (including HIV), and drug-resistant typhoid that have proved astonishingly effective in the resource-poor settings where he works. He is the personification of enhancing the service ethic through action. I used Farmer not only because of what he does but also because of how he deals with it emotionally as well as intellectually. For him, the examined life of serving the disenfranchised is worth living. This inward recognition that Farmer exudes is a prime example of the self-fulfillment that so many of our students were seeking (Eckenfels 1997).

In conjunction with the medical knowledge and organizational skills the students were attaining, the moral development side of the RCSIP experiences prepared them for the reality of life in a world where poverty and discrimination are social facts and one's position in society has a direct influence on one's state of health. By going into these desperately needy communities and serving their populations, the students literally and psychologically stepped outside the taken-for-grant medical world to embrace a set of values that have enduring qualities. Without this kind of clarity, dedication, and feeling of satisfaction, they would simply be learning another set of policies and procedures—perfunctory in nature and repetitious in practice. This is not to put down the rigors of biomedical education and clinical practice. They form the foundation of medical competence. But when this knowledge and its accompanying skills are acquired in a compartmentalized fashion, the emphasis is more on becoming a technician (regardless of how multifaceted) than on being a dedicated and humane practitioner. The intellectual growth and emotional development nurtured through RCSIP involvement was humanistic and moral—the very qualities of a virtuous doctor. A clear sign of this, I believe, is the students' openness in constructing narratives of who they are. It is unequivocally their personal point of view. What better indication of a service ethic is there?

The *community* side of RCSIP involvement provided the students with more than an epidemiological perspective; it allowed them to appreciate the social milieu of the people they were serving. To more fully understand someone, it is necessary to become aware of the particular social and cultural circumstances you find that person in. These experiences tap something elemental—some basic tenet or principle that is at the heart of what medicine is all about in a society concerned with social justice and individual well-being (Soros 2002). It is not enough to obtain medical knowledge and skills; the students, through their own efforts, became socially active and politically aware. The political implications could not be avoided. As Sir Geoffrey Rose (1992), the eminent scholar of social medicine, has proclaimed, "Medicine and politics cannot and should not be kept apart" (129).

I put so much emphasis on the voluntary, student-run aspect of RCSIP because the program is *not* required. Students did it because they felt they had to. They knew that if they didn't do it on their own, it simply would not happen. And they knew it was going to demand a great deal of time and effort. Simply to conceive of such programs as an option goes against conventional thinking in traditional medical education and is therefore considered radical. The formal curriculum of medical training is a series of lessons in detachment and depersonalization that are reinforced most dramatically in the first course in anatomy.

In *The Ethics of Authenticity* (1992), Charles Taylor provides clarity for what I have witnessed among the RCSIP students. In Taylor's terms, idealistic young people today are searching for "horizons of significance" as a source of fulfillment. To reach these goals they need standards of morality to persuade them that their efforts are worthwhile. Much of the ambivalence the medical students feel toward the system under which they are trained comes from the fact that it thwarts authentic development and shrinks from its responsibility to society.

During the decade in which Claudia and I oversaw RCSIP, we were continually amazed at how many faculty and administrators approved of the program without really understanding its implications for the training of future doctors. Very few had the time or inclination to reflect on what the program was promoting. It was outside their fame of reference. The lack of awareness by even those who supported RCSIP was one of the factors that motivated me to write this book. By way of summary this is what they missed:

- If it were a required part of the curriculum, it wouldn't have attracted students seeking a moral purpose.
- The absence of competition played an important role in nurturing the idealism that most students bring to medical school.
- Students (and faculty too) who have tended to keep their humanism to themselves found a group that shares their feelings, representing an opportunity to express these attitudes openly through their actions in serving those outside the system.
- For some ambivalent students RCSIP served as an awakening of the humanistic values that are the core of medicine as a profession.
- By serving poor and disadvantaged people and communities, students developed a sociological awareness of the significance of culture and social class on health and well-being.
- By fostering empathy and sensitivity, the RCSIP participants were able to appreciate the plight of the underprivileged.
- The activist students struggled to ameliorate the feeling of distress that comes from witnessing the sickness and suffering of those who can be helped medically but lack access to health care.
- The ambulatory care the doctors administered was a benefit for the patients and for the community.
- As stated by a group of current RCSIP participants, the major difference between learning clinical concepts and skills in RCSIP and learning them through the preceptorship is that the former allowed them to feel free and collegial with their mentor (making for a better learning environment), whereas the latter was stressful and competitive because they are graded and in competition with their peers for grades.
- Instituting these programs outside the medical center took wisdom, courage, and vision, qualities that give RCSIP its genuineness.

Toward a Humanistic Medical Education

I was never satisfied with merely describing the different projects and their human interest side. I felt a powerful urge to use RCSIP as a catalyst for critically reviewing medicine as a health care practice, an educational environment, and, fundamentally, an institution. My aim was singular: to plant the seeds for change. This gestalt of giving, learning, believing, and acting forms a blueprint for reform in medical education.

To appreciate more fully the potential of RCSIP in this process, I have framed its capacity in terms of three fundamental components: culture, context, and connectedness. From my perspective, it is the integration of culture, as an interrelated pattern of beliefs and predispositions, with the context of structural factors such as social status, resource availability, and political power—in other words, how core values interact with a social structure—that can form the basis of a more encompassing health policy. Such a policy is necessary for spurring a renewal of the public trust that is required to reconnect medicine to society. From a pedagogical perspective, my aim is to show that an understanding and application of these social phenomena enhance the maturation of humanistic physicians dedicated to ensuring quality care and promoting sustainable health. In short, reforming medicine requires reframing medical education.

Culture

Culture is difficult to explain concretely because it is amorphous, diffuse, and elusive. It is also ubiquitous and all encompassing. Today, there is a culture of everything, but most discussions of culture lack substance and are merely rhetorical devices. For my thesis, however, culture has particular meaning not only because it is basic to understanding all social phenomena, but, in particular, because it is relevant to medicine's moral imperative to train socially responsible physicians capable of providing affordable, safe, and accessible health care to a rapidly changing and culturally diversified society (and, for that matter, world). In other words, I need to address how the individual internalizes culture (Ortner 2006) "without losing sight of the larger structures that constrain (but also enable) social action" (3). To illustrate this, I look at culture in two distinct ways: first, how it is taught in medical school, the all-encompassing nature of medical school culture, and the culture unique to RCSIP, and, second, the cultural tensions that are emerging in our ethnic and racially diverse society and that challenge what Tocqueville described as "habits of the heart," an expression of the mixture of mores and traits that constitute our "national character."

Denise Wear (2003) presents an excellent analysis of the way culture is misunderstood in medical education and how this misunderstanding actually leads to potentially harmful attitudes and stereotyping of "others" from different racial, ethnic, and social groups. The thrust of her argument is based on Giroux's (2000) concept of *insurgent multiculturalism,* which lends credence to my own concerns about the nexus of social responsibility and duty. When it comes to the "culture issues," medical educators argue that they have addressed the situation by instituting courses in cultural competency, which, as Wear points out, are "sometimes known as cultural sensitivity, cultural awareness, or simply multi-culturalism" (549). Like their counterpart in medical ethics, such courses focus on learning specific characteristics of various "ethnic groups" lumped together and viewed as one inevitable identity. The idea of culture as dynamic and fluid is never considered. In fact, the immutability of culture is the premise on which cultural competency is based. In a course on social medicine that I directed, a Latino student, regarding certain dietary habits of Mexican Americans, com-mented, "They act as if we don't like Chinese food." Cultural considerations in medical ethics are all about the doctor-patient relationship and its ethical and legal ramifications, primarily for the health care provider. In this process, cul-ture becomes medicalized. Although inequalities among certain segments of society may be identified, the source of those inequalities is never discussed. I once asked the faculty who taught bioethics at Rush how they dealt with social injustice. The answer was a chilling silence.

Wear again turns to the radical pedagogy of Giroux to demonstrate the sig-nificance of insurgent multiculturalism. In fact, according to Giroux, attention must be shifted "away from an exclusive focus on subordinated groups, espe-cially since such an approach tends to highlight their deficits, to one that exam-ines how racism [and other expressions of dominance and neglect] in its various forms is produced historically, semiotically, and institutionally at vari-ous levels of society" (Wear 2003, 551). What is especially important about this comment is that RCSIP participants came face to face with these conditions. Wear goes on to say that if an insurgent multiculturalism is used as a moral underpinning of a social medicine curricular component, "students would have opportunities to learn and practice the skills of critical analysis to identify the inequalities and injustices within the doctor-patient relationship, medical education and teaching hospitals, and health care access and delivery in the United States" (552). She further warns, and I have learned from experience, that such an epiphany does not occur from a one-shot deal, a well-taught course, a moving lecture, or a mission statement. To be effective, such experi-ences and their reflective appreciation need to be firmly anchored in longitudi-nal activities that are built upon and internalized, that is, a process that promotes moral behavior through learning how to act rather than what to think.

In the broadest sense, understanding culture as a concept is necessary for grasping the vast diversity that our society has embraced.

Understanding how the culture of the medical school influences the learning and development of future physicians is essential for any proposed change. As mentioned in the introduction, Hafferty and Franks (1994) have distinguished three different curricula, namely, the formal curriculum, as described in academic medical center mission statements; the informal curriculum, done through individual mentoring and examples; and the hidden curriculum, the lessons about how to achieve success, taught behind the scenes. Hafferty's original curricula provide a valuable construct for framing the structure of contemporary American medical education. He is especially astute at recognizing and defining the social order and how future physicians are socialized from matriculation to graduation and beyond.

In my discussions with Hafferty, I proposed a fourth curriculum, the peripheral curriculum, or voluntary community service, in which moral principles and personal development are being advanced through direct action and personal commitment. Building on his conceptual scheme, I have tried to go a step further by addressing a concern about the cultural configurations that constitute medical education. Change cannot be instituted in these structures unless the mores, customs, rituals, and role identifications associated with them are acknowledged. In totality, RCSIP is more than a peripheral curriculum; it is a *subculture* with distinct values, attitudes and beliefs, and clearly discernible patterns of personal and social action. This subculture was born in response to the mainstream culture of contemporary medical education, with its emphasis on retention of facts, subservience to hierarchical authority, and detached practice procedures that reflect a reliance on costly new technology and an acceptance of a business protocol.

An awareness of these conditions was the main reason the students started RCSIP. Ironically, the small introduction to social and cultural factors in my community health course served as a catalyst for bringing personal discontent about these conditions to a collective concern. It created a common bond that the concerned students had not known was possible. Most important, they wanted and got an opportunity to act on their idealism. As the students have stated repeatedly in their narratives, following their exposure to poor and inner-city communities, they hoped to continue these experiences in residency programs and practice settings that were not solely centered in the academic health center.

Actually, it is more accurate to say the students formed a *counterculture*—a system of beliefs and actions that was counter to the education of the modern physician as technician and provider of a market product. The structure of

RCSIP—duties and responsibilities, scheduling of assignments, logistical operations, design and institution of projects—was sustained by the humanism the
original organizers shared. Their narratives are replete with statements of satisfaction gained from RCSIP participation as compared with the effects of formal
medical college courses and rotations. In his critique of efforts to reform the
medical school curriculum, Hafferty (1998) has proposed that medical school
be thought of as a "learning environment" and that reform initiatives be undertaken on the basis of what students learn rather than on what they are taught.
He has said that "the very work of developing, implementing, and evaluating
[a new curriculum] conveys to faculty and students alike a variety of messages
about what is and what should be valued within the community" (404). In fact,
he contends that the existing culture of medical education, with its ambiguous
ethical principles, has spawned the hidden curriculum as a form of adaptation.
Benevolence, altruism, humanitarianism, and dutifulness are supposed to be
the underlying values that justify, on moral grounds, the biomedical knowledge
and skills that serve as the basis for caring. Medicine, traditionally, is very
moralistic in the "doctor knows best" sense. A contemporary example is the
obsession with "lifestyle interventions." The health professional knows what is
best for you. Professionalism for professionalism's sake will not fill the gap.

From a societal viewpoint, understanding the "stuff of culture" is absolutely
necessary to seeing how culturally derived attitudes and beliefs affect the
health and well-being of people from different cultural backgrounds. But
understanding the various subcultures found in the contemporary United
States is very deceiving. African Americans, who did not come here willingly,
have a special significance in this mosaic. Their status, as one side of the color
line (Du Bois 1903), serves to sustain what Orlando Patterson (2006) so astutely
observes is "the segregation of blacks from the social, communal, and intimate
cultural life of white Americans."

There is also the vast array of "new cultures" brought by immigrants who
have arrived from Cambodia, Laos, and Thailand in Southeastern Asia; Middle
Easterners from places like Pakistan, Iran, Lebanon, and Syria; sub-Saharan
Africans; and indigenous peoples of Central and South America. Many of these
people, like those served by Casa Guatemala, came to the United States as
political refugees seeking sanctuary. And there are the more established
(Americanized) subcultures of the second half of the twentieth century such
as Mexican Americans, Puerto Ricans, Indians, and Japanese. These more
ensconced immigrant groups, many of them now third generation, have been
well acculturated to "the American way of life" as depicted in the media or
passed on through their children's peer groups in school. But how they have

adapted to the complexities of this country depends on many factors, such as how long they remain in the subculture of an ethnic community and what kinds of opportunities they have had with respect to education and work. The situation is further complicated by the political firestorm caused by the situation of undocumented immigrants crossing the border from Mexico. In the 1960s, when I first studied American culture, the post–melting pot conceptualization was cultural pluralism. The beauty of this concept for democracy was the coexistence of one's roots with a unique American character. Religious beliefs were an accepted part of the original cultural background. The Italians who celebrate the Feast of San Gennaro in New York City are loyal and patriotic Americans.

There are numerous paradoxes about culture in this country. An excellent example of this can be found in Ann Fadiman's *The Spirit Catches You and You Fall Down* (1997), the moving account of Lia Lee, a Hmong child with epilepsy, and the American doctors who try to care for her. It is an amazing description of confrontation between two cultures and its devastating effects. The physicians are accustomed to giving orders based on accepted "physicians' authority" but find this attitude futile when they run up against the stubborn Hmong character that for millennia preferred death to surrender. This poignant story demonstrates how the two cultures, one of spirituality based on kinship and the other of medicine based on science, never really find common ground for compromise, mutual trust, and understanding. These kinds of tensions are commonplace for anthropologists in their search for answers to basic questions pertaining to human nature.

In a marvelous book, *Why America's Top Pundits Are Wrong: Anthropologists Talk Back* (2005), Besteman and Gusterson list in their introduction a "loosely coherent set of myths about human nature and culture that have strong staying power in American public discourse" (2) such as the notions "that conflict between people of different cultures, races, or gender is inevitable; that biology is destiny; that culture is immutable; that terrible poverty, inequality, and suffering are natural; and that people in other societies who don't want to live just like Americans are afraid of 'modernity'" (2). The action taken by the RCSIP participants at the community and grassroots levels exposed them to these conditions. Moreover, this exposure made them sensitive to the value system of those they were serving, resulting in a more compassionate perspective, in contrast to the detached, reductive, procedural one they were accustomed to. In sum, this immersion in minority, poor, disadvantaged communities was an antidote to the misinterpretation and misuse of culture found in the conventional wisdom of standard American medical education.

If real reform is to take place from within medicine, then it is absolutely essential to learn the covert aspects of medical education and their powerful effect on how doctors are socialized to the profession. Attributes such as altruism and empathy that are espoused as the core values become displaced throughout medical training. The students' first patients—the cadavers in anatomy—are about as depersonalized as you can get. A business culture, couched in terms of the bottom line, has taken precedence over a humanistic one. In addition, culture, as a component of a person's state of well-being, is left out of a biomedical model that is firmly anchored in the doctor-patient relationship centering on diagnosis and treatment. Furthermore, the culture of medical education tends to be highly compartmentalized, with each component following the previous one in lockstep fashion. Order within academic medicine is maintained traditionally by a hierarchy of position and power that is rigorously adhered to. This is the acculturation that is dominant in the current professionalization of medicine. Moreover, some who hold more dominant positions in the hierarchy fear that medicine is losing its professional status. In the vein of health services research, the emphasis on quantification leaves culture out of almost every assessment of health care because it cannot be measured statistically. Whether it is a clinical trial, a program evaluation, or an analysis of quality care, the methodology is considered meaningless unless it is based on quantifiable outcomes. In fact, culture is absent from the evidence-based medicine and information network paradigms. Translational research seems to be more content in leaving it out as well.[2]

Richard Rorty, the distinguished social philosopher of the late twentieth century, encouraged my thinking in this regard through the stated goal of creating "a greater diversity of individuals—larger, fuller, and more imaginative and daring individuals." "Individual life will become unthinkably diverse and social life unthinkably free" (Brooks 2007). I firmly believe that if modern medicine is to make its contribution, to paraphrase Rorty (1997), "achieving our diversified society," it must embrace the power of culture—intellectually, emotionally, and morally. Without an understanding and appreciation of culture there are no socially centered projects to propose for promoting health and well-being, no vision of a humanistic profession committed to service, and no idealistic physicians for building a consensus on the need for specific reforms.

Context

From what I've said so far, it should be clear that it is really impossible to separate culture from structure; nonetheless, since culture is so pervasive and amorphous, it still needs a discernible context that gives it substance and meaning, that is, something you can get a handle on. Any proposed reform in medical education based on principles garnered from the RCSIP experience must be set in a social structure with specific reference to social status and the factors that determine it. Context is the structural framework in which cultural conflicts occur. This is particularly relevant today because there is growing controversy about "diversity" and "social class." Diversity gained prominence in medical school admissions following the Supreme Court's ruling in *Bakke v. Board of Regents,* 1978, which said that the University of California could, "as part of its legitimate interest in maintaining a diverse student body, take race into account when admitting students." Walter Benn Michaels, in his most recent book, *The Trouble with Diversity* (2007), asks us to consider the harm done when we worry about identity and forget about inequality. I believe that this is not an either/or proposition. It is the convergence of culture, race, and ethnicity with the social hierarchy of status and position that provides a much better basis for understanding and addressing the issue of health care disparities. If the contemporary physician is dedicated to alleviating sickness and suffering in the patient, then he or she must be able to recognize it in the family, the neighborhood, the community, and society. The reciprocal relationship between health and poverty is well established. But the diversity must be addressed as well. For me, Kerr White's (1991) *health care ecology model* provides the handle for seeing how culture and class interact and are distributed in time and place.

Michael Marmot (2004) has demonstrated through decades of carefully conducted empirical research that "as bad as poverty is for health, what is really at issue here is inequality" (240). He calls this phenomenon "the status syndrome." "All societies," he writes, "have rankings because individuals are unequal in a variety of ways; but not all societies have the same gradient in health. What matters is the degree to which inequalities in ranking lead to inequalities in capabilities—being able to lead the lives they most want to lead. Central to these capabilities are autonomy and social participation." He goes on to say, "Control over one's life and opportunities for meaningful social engagement are necessary for health. It is also likely the relationship goes the other way: without good health it is hard to achieve autonomy and full social engagement" (241). Implicit in Marmot's analysis are the cultural constraints that limit capabilities. If you live in a poor black or Latino community, your identity has a strong effect on your autonomy, how you are perceived, and your participation outside your own ethnic or racial group.

Medical students are given very little training in the significance of the social context and its role in identifying determinants of health and illness. In a social-epidemiology assessment, for example, social class pertains to education, occupation, and income; these categories, along with others such as age, gender, and ethnicity, can be quantified, classified, or both, for correlation purposes to pinpoint a particular phenomenon such as diabetes. It is obviously important to know that young black men have the highest rate of type II diabetes, but because of measurement limitations the explanation ends there. Members of minority groups are not classifications and numbers; they are individuals with lives and meaning. These analytical categories are considered objective but, regardless, are also cross-sectional points in time (U.S. census data) and in no way represent the fluidity of income and occupation that is prevalent in our society.

There are many examples of this social context that resonate. The struggle of the working poor is vividly depicted by Barbara Ehrenreich in *Nickel and Dimed* (2001). To survive a day, let alone a lifetime, with the realization of how quickly aspirations fade is heartbreaking. This struggle is either completely ignored or accepted as appropriate in corporate America. The end of welfare as we know it certainly hasn't improved the lot of those trapped in dead-end jobs.

As Sharon Cohen (2005) reports, the lot of the homeless has become especially disturbing. Although a recent Associated Press poll found that 53 percent of Americans consider homelessness a very serious problem, the homeless have become Ralph Ellison's proverbial "invisible man," that is, we don't see them anymore and, if we do, we ignore them. Cohen sums up her snapshots of the homeless thus: "From villages to large cities, homelessness has spread like dye through the weave of America's social fabric. A single day in the life of the homeless reveals hundreds of thousands without shelter, and blame goes to everything from the lack of affordable housing and unemployment to drug abuse, mental illness and a flawed foster care system." Rush students not only see them but also serve them in several shelters where they volunteer.

Oscar Lewis (2002), as participant-observer in Mexican ghettos, characterized the conditions he saw as a "culture of poverty." David Shipler stated in an op-ed piece in the *New York Times* (2004a) that poverty is "more like an ecological system of relationships among individuals, families, and the environment of schools, neighborhoods, jobs, and government services." Shipler has written a disquieting book, *The Working Poor* (2004b), which is about the people who are not making it in the same America where CEOs make four hundred times what their average worker makes. Shipler's book is especially meaningful because of its insight into the tangled web of job discrimination, bureaucratic red tape, and unhealthy living conditions that keep the poor, even those who work full time, trapped in what Shipler calls "the insidious, self-reinforcing nature of poverty." These conditions, pervasive in poor, minority, urban communities occupied by those individuals that Wilson (1987) refers to as the "truly disadvantaged," are the substance of the world where RCSIP intervenes.

Urban poor black communities, like Henry Horner Homes, seem to be especially unhealthy. We are not talking about infectious diseases such as sexually
transmitted diseases, tuberculosis, or AIDS, although they do exist at higher-
than-average rates. We are talking about chronic diseases such as stroke, diabetes, hypertension, kidney failure, and certain types of cancer. Helen Epstein
(2003) documents that "some of these neighborhoods have the highest mortality rates in the country, but this is not, as many believe, mainly because of drug
overdoses and gunshot wounds." In her article, Epstein uses the term *miasma,*
which seems to provide a fitting metaphor for this new epidemic of chronic disease concentrated in poor, minority urban neighborhoods.

Everywhere in Horner we discovered roach dust, a major trigger for
asthma. Studies have shown that childhood asthma rates drop dramatically
when the children's families move to better communities (Weiss, Gergen, and
Hodgson 1992). In my course on community health, I had the students do an
ecological assessment (a windshield survey) of the urban neighborhoods they
visited. They found vacant lots; boarded-up buildings; advertisements for ciga-
rettes and alcohol; and an absence of parks, playgrounds, grass, and trees. In
our asthma project we found that many mothers, through fear of gang violence
and drug dealing, kept their children indoors. In the context of life in the projects, the students witnessed the interplay of aspirations, hope, and spirit with
anger, hostility, and despair.

Robert Putman (2000) found that the decline of social capital—the capacity of the group to bind people together by sharing common interests that are for
the betterment of the individual members as well as the group—turned out to
be clearly correlated with diminished safety and increased crime, heightened
risk to children's welfare, impaired economic efficiency, alarming drops in
public health, and a shortened lifespan.

Besides the poverty and deprivation they saw, the message that came
through loud and clear to the student volunteers was the inequality and injustice of it all. In a course in epidemiology or public health, students may hear
about the growing number of disadvantaged people in the United States, but
numbers don't make minorities; it is how people are treated that makes minorities. Only experiential learning awakens students to this tragedy.

Epstein (2003) provides evidence for both environmental and psychological stress factors in the incidence of chronic disease among the urban poor.
Other observers corroborate her notion that hopelessness and depression are
significant for understanding what is at stake. What is needed is a renewed
sense of hope and possibility. RCSIP participants saw these conditions firsthand, not only in terms of housing and income (or lack of them), but as what

Nussbaum (2001) calls "upheavals of thought," those feelings that portend emotional states and a sense of self and family manifested in their daily lives.

Two narratives by student activists add the highly personal touch of what I mean. Peter DeGolia's account of a particular patient encounter paints a vivid picture of what the attributes cultivated through active RCSIP participation meant to him as a geriatrician practicing in a poor neighborhood of Cleveland. (Since the time he related this story, he has become the director of the Center on Geriatric Medicine at University Hospitals, Case Medical Center.)

Every Thursday afternoon Mrs. Tucker and I made home visits together. She was a nurse from Senior Services, and I was, and still am, an attending physician in the Department of Family Medicine at MetroHealth, the large county medical center located in Cleveland, Ohio. I provided home care to homebound older adults in a medically underserved and impoverished neighborhood on Cleveland's East Side in the shadow of the Cleveland Clinic Foundation. On this day we were performing a follow-up visit to see Mrs. J, a morbidly obese African American woman who owned her own dilapidated home two blocks from one of the worst public housing projects in the city. Several months earlier I became her primary care physician. She had not seen a doctor in nearly two years. The community social service agency was concerned about her lack of medical care and suspicious that her caregiver was involved in financial abuse. She was initially "cared for" by a former nurse's aide, a white woman from the nearby suburb of Shaker Heights, who had befriended her years earlier and subsequently came to control her finances. At the time I became involved, the nurse's aide no longer provided direct personal care. She had arranged for the Area Agency on Aging to provide the personal health care services. While it may seem insignificant, Mrs. J's income amounted to over $2,000 per month from her pension and social security. I was assigned to determine her health and well-being. My first task was to better understand if she was clinically competent to make self-care decisions.

Mrs. J was bed bound due to her morbid obesity and arthritis. She had a body shaped like a pancake with a small head that would rotate thirty degrees right and left and arms that moved. At first she seemed cognitively appropriate and had adapted to her living situation by devising a network of ropes that, when pulled, would turn a light and a fan on and off and open and close her front door. Her bed was positioned in the large front room with a picture window where she could see who was coming and going. Mrs. J made a habit of befriending those less fortunate than herself. She had a "son" who lived with her that I learned later was a young man she had befriended and offered a place to live. She felt that he provided security for her.

Her food was purchased weekly by the caregiver (nurse's aide), who also paid her bills and arranged for her health care, which, prior to my involvement, consisted of being seen at a local community hospital by an acute-care physician her caregiver knew personally. At this time I determined that Mrs. J was not capable of making self-care decisions. Through intimidation or habit, she deferred all decisions to her caregiver. As I investigated the situation more closely, I began to question the safety and appropriateness of Mrs. J's living conditions. The more I questioned the situation the more I met resistance by the caregiver.

On the day Mrs. Tucker and I showed up to make our final assessment, we were met by a drunk and hostile "son." In an "in my face" confrontation, he threatened to seriously harm me if I moved his "mother out of our house." With Mrs. Tucker trying desperately to calm him down, we edged our way toward the front door. Mrs. J was oblivious to the interaction or implications before her.

We learned a hard lesson that day. We had been "set up" by the Shaker Heights caregiver. She had told this man that if I determined Mrs. J to be clinically incompetent and obtained a court-appointed guardian, she would be moved out of her home and he would be out on the street. His arrangement of a free place to live and her arrangement of significant income would come crashing down. What they anticipated, of course, happened.

As I reflect on that particular episode and why I stayed the course (despite threats to my life), I see a chain of events, contemplations, introspections (whatever you like) leading up to it. I also see a personal motivation (probably instilled early in my life) and the numerous decisions (including some very poor ones) in hopes of keeping it alive. When it comes to my vocation, medicine, certain milestones come to mind. When I read the narratives of my fellow RCSIP activists, I see myself more vividly and the many good fortunes, as well as difficulties, I have experienced in my professional education and development. But what especially stands out is the opportunity to have these attitudes and beliefs reaffirmed and reinforced by the role I played in the creation and implementation of the Rush Community Service Initiatives Program early in my training at Rush. I would like now to offer a capsule version of that involvement.

Now, fourteen years after graduation from Rush Medical College, I remain engaged in social justice and the fight against inequality. I am

trained as a family physician and geriatrician working for the
MetroHealth System, a well-run, safety net, public health system of
Cuyahoga County, Ohio. My professional responsibilities include direct
clinical care to vulnerable older adults throughout the service area and
in some county nursing homes, as well as administrative responsibility
for post-acute-care services within the MetroHealth System. My work
offers me a unique blend between social activism and direct service.

Peter has come back to Chicago on many occasions since his graduation from
Rush. He has talked to current RCSIP participants about what the program fostered for him and his career choice in medicine. They sit enthralled, listening
to someone who really practices what he believes in.

Michelle Bardack, a family practice doctor, has returned to her love of caring for Native Americans and other community people in New Mexico. Before
she left after a few years' stay in Chicago, she told me this story:

Earlier this fall I was sitting at my local library in the "quiet" room. In
trudged a handsome young man with a large backpack of books and a
look of gloom on his face. As he slumped into his chair, I recognized one
of the books he piled up high beside him. "Excuse me, are you a medical
student?" I asked. "Yah," he answered exhaustedly. From this introduction a long discussion followed in which he shared with me how miser-
able he was just going to lectures taking notes, taking tests. He ultimately
quit going to classes and just studied in the library 24–7 and showed up
at school for the tests. That was his medical school experience for two
years. And he was thinking of dropping out because he was so disgusted.
I shared with him my experiences at St. Basil's and in RCSIP, and asked
if his school offered anything like that. He let out a laugh of irony and
said, "No way. Too much work, no one would want to do that." It made
me sad because this kid seemed so burned out as a medical student, I
just wondered what might happen to him in the future.

I realized that because of what Ed and Claudia offered to me with RCSIP,
I entered medicine with a passion; it was nurtured in these programs and I
am now out practicing still with this passionate altruistic heart that Ed and
Claudia would not let traditional training extinguish in me.

What Michelle is expressing most is her feelings about what being a doctor
means to her. This interest in her patients and the community she serves transcend her clinical competence and authenticates her purpose for wanting to
become a doctor in the first place.

Peter's and Michelle's narratives offer a snapshot of how they grasp the fullness of their lives as health care providers. There is no separation from being caring doctors and concerned persons. Their perception of who they are is an extension of what they do. Their account of these two incidents—one a manipulated disabled person, the other a disillusioned student—are not cursory descriptions, but, instead, something fundamentally human that requires wisdom and empathy.

Connectedness

As one of our society's major institutions, medicine is a product of that society. The two are intractably intertwined and cannot be separated. Without healthy members, society is diminished; without societal support, medicine is useless. But, as I have argued, medicine, as a compassionate and healing art, has become disconnected from society. Before medicine can reconnect, it must become cognizant of the society of which it is an integral part. However, it has tried to keep pace with rapid changes of modernity by emulating the technological and instrumental developments and disregarding cultural, social, and political movements. The assumption is that the continued growth of procedural and technical advances will, through the ingenuity of these advances, improve the care and cure of the sick and suffering. This has proved true for particular illnesses and specific patients. But, despite these incredibly costly advances, dangers lurk in the procedures themselves, personal dissatisfaction with quality of care continues to rise, the lack of accessibility to medical services for millions is not remedied, and the overall health of our society has not shown discernible improvement, particularly when it is compared with other countries.

As mentioned in the introduction, there has been a plethora of reports that look to professionalism as the magic bullet that will restore medicine to its former esteemed status. The accepted modus operandi, first stated by the Cruesses (Cruess and Cruess 1997), for initiating and sustaining this renewing professionalism is through a revised medical education curriculum with integrated courses geared toward the advancement of professionalism. Some critics (Hafferty 2000) do not accept this strategy, since contemporary medicine has by design excluded professionalism as the core of medical training and replaced it with a heavy emphasis on technical knowledge and skills. Wear and Castellani (2000) believe that a full-spectrum curriculum, not just another course in medical ethics, is needed to foster professional attitudes and values in future physicians. Although Freidson's (1987) sociological conceptualization (a unique body of knowledge and skills and control of the teaching and certification of future doctors) has been the accepted framework for defining medicine as a profession, it is essentially static with respect to dynamic social forces. In addition, it leaves out the historical roots of medicine as a profession as distinguished from being a trade, that is, why certain forms of work were given this special status.

Professionalism is the elephant in the room, and like Lakoff's (2004) students, medicine cannot stop thinking about it. I believe that the intrinsic values of medicine must be reframed not simply as an exercise in rhetoric but as the very essence of medicine's fiduciary responsibility to society. Keep in mind that practically every form of work in our society is considered a profession today, from plumbing to garbage collection (now done by a "sanitation engineer"). Athletes and entertainers (rock stars, in particular) have pushed to be perceived as professionals. But there is a strong negative connotation to this use of professionalism. Many "professional" athletes are seen as too rich, self-centered, spoiled, and involved frequently in such dangerous behavior as fights, rape, drug use, and even murder. Emphasizing medicine as a profession doesn't automatically guarantee the return of its prestige and privilege.

I have also found that altruism and dutifulness, as the moral imperatives of academic medicine (MSOP 1998), do not sit well with medical students. If you are Mother Teresa or Paul Farmer (whom the students admire more than anyone else in health care), altruism seems natural. But if you graduate from medical school $150,000 or more in debt, want to start a family and pursue a worthwhile career, you are under great pressures simply to survive. Moreover, my experience is that students resent the notion of dutifulness. They see it as a form of conscription and it dampens any social motivation they may have been trying to nurture.

The confluence of culture, as a system of values and beliefs, and the social context, as a stratification system of status and opportunity, shapes attitudes and behaviors and creates the structure for social behavior. An understanding of this interrelationship offers an intellectual and moral basis for creating just and humane health care. These are also fundamental constructs for designing and executing a humanistic and sociocultural medical education. But, in conjunction with educational reform, a feasible plan is also needed for restoring the ethical underpinnings of medicine as a *practice* that has become dominated by forms of cost-benefit analysis and specialty procedures that often sideline the kind of care that involves treating the patient as a whole person with a life story and not as just the locus of a technical problem.

Nonetheless, in the current evidence-based and information-network environment, medical practice is confronted with multiple paradoxes. As practitioners become immersed in expanding new technology, they slowly, and in many cases unwittingly, give up their humanity. This is not to suggest that they become automatons, but rather to note that they are compelled by the forces within medicine to use the tools science has provided them, too often, to the exclusion of social and cultural factors and their influence on how illness and disease are perceived by the individual, the community, and society. On another level, and in some ways more pervasively, becoming a physician is to become engulfed in competition and commercialism. In short, today's young doctors are faced with agonizing contradictions that overwhelm them.

Fortunately, the conspiracy of silence that has shrouded medicine's objectionable side is now being exposed. The pharmaceutical industry has inadvertently revealed its profit motive, which has contaminated the ethics of clinical research (Angel 2004). High infection rates, with mortality at 15 percent, have become the scourge of hospitals (Connolly 2005). Iatrogenic disease has made patients fearful of being hospitalized. In *How Doctors Think,* Jerome Groopman (2007) takes great care to emphasize the importance of doctors recognizing their mistakes and the need to disseminate information on rates of errors not only to the medical profession, but to the patient as well. The preconditions for instituting real change are there.

Corporatization, commodification, and instrumentalization have driven medicine away from its inherent purpose—the prime responsibility of looking after the health and well-being of all members of society. This call of service has been the wellspring of medicine since Hippocrates. Instead of putting so much weight on professionalism as a privileged status (many students see the white-coat ceremony in this light), medicine would do better to enhance the idealism of most young people who want to be physicians so they can look after people, rather than burning it out of them by focusing exclusively on procedures and techniques. Companion to this idealism is the cultivation of a humanism that nurtures empathy, sensitivity, and other values. What I am proposing is not just a change in terminology but a revival of moral principles.

This is where RCSIP fits in. It was not a passing fancy for those truly committed individuals who were willing to invest so much of themselves in making it a reality. I believe that those students recognized early in their medical education that something absolutely fundamental had been left out, not in technical skills or scientific and biomedical knowledge, but in a moral sense. For them, medicine was, and will continue to be, more a vocation than a profession. They certainly want to become the most competent physicians possible, but that is a means, not an end in itself. The competent doctor is also the *good* doctor.

Garry Wills's (2000) keen observations about why there has been a dearth of religious vocations among idealistic young Catholics parallel my own observations regarding RCSIP participants. Into Wills's comments, I add my interjections: "Young idealistic persons, the kind who want to be priests [doctors], are just the people for whom matters of honesty with themselves are bound to be most challenging. How can one aspire to a high calling and yet accept low standards for his own truthfulness about what he really believes? How can one be in service to others, yet peddle to them religious truths [professional standards] whose truthfulness rings so obviously hollow?" (5).

The narratives of students still in medical school and those of practicing doctors echo Wills's point. The struggle just below the surface, Hafferty's (1994) hidden curriculum, continues to be buried. The professional side of medicine cannot deal with it regardless of how many reports are written, how many talks are given, and how many committees are formed to look into it.

More than anything else, RCSIP should give all of us hope through the actions and sense of responsibility it promotes. These experiences do not take place in a vacuum. Any reflection on them, especially among idealistic and bright young people, results in placing the activities in a broader social context. They become aware of and are directed toward facing the health care issues I raised earlier. Moreover, RCSIP participation operates as a centrifugal force, drawing interested, inquisitive, and often confused medical students into a world, a culture, a value system, a moral order that taxes their intellect, tests their will, and bonds them with others of similar attitudes and beliefs. RCSIP is not just another fascinating extracurricular venture, but an obsession of sorts that binds together the emotional and intellectual demands of physicians in training with the ability to become part of something much bigger. In short, they have found their own authenticity by recognizing the humanity of others.

If it were a required part of the curriculum, it would not affect the students in the same way. To make participation mandatory would defeat the altruistic motivation of those who want to volunteer and introduce the negative attitudes of those who don't but are forced into it. The absence of competition plays an important role in encouraging the optimism most students bring to medical school. The motivation of the activist students illustrates Paul Farmer's awareness of the need to ameliorate the distress that comes from witnessing sickness and the suffering of those who can be helped medically.

Claudia and I have repeatedly heard students voice the ambivalence of which Farmer speaks. I actually think it is more difficult for the students. They have not mapped out their careers yet, but they are pulled in many different directions at once. Their questions reveal deeply felt concerns: How can I keep this commitment alive? Where do I go for residency training? Where will I practice? How can I make a difference as well as make a living? Of course, all medical students ask these same questions as they approach graduation. But for the RCSIP participants it is more than a job (profession); it is humanistic medicine.

Keep in mind that RCSIP was started by students who put themselves on the line to make it work. It continues to evolve on its own. It provides needed services to the poor and disadvantaged. It creates a milieu for breeding humanism. It encourages participants to become sensitive to the plight of the disenfranchised. It fosters a sense of responsibility for those in need. It facilitates an ability to become an advocate for social justice and human rights. In sum, it strives, through its action, to reconnect medicine to society.

Medical Education Reform as a Catalyst for Change

In addition to promoting culture and social context (as I have described them) as essential components for reforming medical education, my assessment must recognize the effect of specific factors external to medicine's core values such as escalating costs, limited access, and the declining perception of quality of health care if my argument is to have merit. Following this line of reasoning, I believe that if medical education is the point of reform in medicine, it must be recast to meet challenges from the growing concern for some form of universal health care, give serious consideration to the value of prevention both for promoting health and as a cost-effective measure, and respond to the urgent need for generalist physicians to provide community-based health care for the millions of uninsured. With respect to the last point, there is a growing shortage of health personnel that is not restricted to doctors and nurses but extends to a broad spectrum of allied health workers. The situation is further exacerbated by the dearth of members of minority groups in medicine and the lack of any discernible program to recruit and retain them.

Universal Health Care

Some form of universal health care is on the horizon. (Because it is an issue that requires a book in its own right, I will try to keep to the points that are salient to my position.) In February 2003, Representative John Conyers Jr. unveiled a bill, the United States National Health Insurance Act (HR 676), that would establish a single-payer national health program. The emphasis on single-payer has been central to the mission of the group Physicians for a National Health Program (PNHP). Until recently, health care reform has taken a backseat to the war in Iraq. However, it is once again rising to the surface as a serious issue on the minds of most Americans.

All the presidential candidates have had to come up with some kind of health care plan. But universal health care entails as many interpretations as it does proposals. State plans in California and Massachusetts have received a lot of attention. These state proposals, regardless of their shortcomings, appear to

be on a collision course with the Bush administration's plan of establishing
health accounts. An additional $12 billion over five years in annual funds for
the State Children's Health Insurance Plan (SCHIP) and Medicaid would allow
the enrollment of most of the uninsured children already eligible for the program.[3] At the time of this writing, a coalition of fifty-five organizations has sent
a letter to Congress asking for this funding. The *Christian Science Monitor*
wrote an editorial highlighting that Wal-Mart and the Service Employees
International Union (SEIU) have launched a proposal with the goal of affordable health care for all U.S. residents by 2012. Don McCanne (2007) of PNHP
believes that "the new insurance mandates [of these programs] will hand [the
private health insurance firms] billions in wasteful administrative fees that do
not occur in government insurance programs such as Medicare." "Medicare for
all" has become the battle cry for a score of nonprofit organizations working on
health care reform. Jacob Hacker, of the Brookings Institution, has proposed
universal insurance to enhance economic security and to promote opportunity.
Universal health care has become a favorite topic in Paul Krugman's *New York
Times* columns. John Edwards has made it a high priority in his presidential
campaign. Paul Krugman (2007a) has called Edwards's plan "a smart, serious
proposal [that] addresses both the problem of the uninsured and the waste and
inefficiency of our fragmented insurance system." It has become commonplace
for health care reform critics to blame uncontrolled costs on the pharmaceutical industry and insurance companies, which continue to generate huge prof-
its. The Veterans Administration's medical care system has been cited as a
paragon of cost-effective, quality, comprehensive care. (This was prior to the
Walter Reed Hospital fiasco that occurred under privatized care.) Lake Research
Partners, a nonprofit health care research group, has proposed calling universal
health care "quality, affordable health care."[4]

A main source of conflict within the health-care-for-all contingent is the clash
between the public and private sectors. The Bush administration's major thrust for
reform entails privatization. A good example is Medicare Part D. As Krugman
(2007b) explains: "There's no traditional Medicare version of Part D, in which the
government pays drug costs directly. Instead, the elderly must get coverage from a
private insurance company, which then receives a government subsidy." In addition, the "doughnut hole," that is, cessation of coverage when a specific cost level
is reached, is extremely confusing and, for many elderly, a financial shock. An
even more insidious result of the federal government's affair with privatizing is
the unwillingness of the Department of Health and Human Services to buy for-
mulary drugs in bulk at a much cheaper price, which leaves the individual with
the responsibility to purchase the prescriptions at a very high cost.

Finding a fiscal solution to universal health care is a daunting task. Unfortunately, most Americans don't believe it can be done. Arnold Relman (2007), a former editor of the *New England Journal of Medicine,* tags some of the obstacles, such as fee-for-service payments of physicians, investor-owned facilities, and a market ideology that would have to be replaced by salaried physicians working in prepaid medical groups and by nonprofit ownership. A difficult agenda, but nothing less will do. David Himmelstein and Steffie Woolhandler, founders of PNHP, are critical of both Krugman and Edwards on a number of fronts. Nevertheless, some form of universal health care is no longer a speck on the horizon but is now a ship in the harbor. As Ed O'Neil (2007), director of the Center for the Health Professions, says, however, "We should closely examine the true nature of the needs before we build the new capacity-generating resource."

Prevention

Regardless of what form this movement toward universal health care takes, prevention will be at the heart of any and all interventions. This is not only because it improves the health of everyone, but also because it is cost-effective. Of all the aspects of health care, prevention is the least emphasized. Millions are missing out on preventive health screening for cancer, asthma, diabetes, and AIDS. In this era of chronic diseases, this is more than discouraging; it is unconscionable. This is particularly true for the poor and disadvantaged and the rest of the uninsured. Race and ethnicity correlate significantly with higher rates of common chronic illnesses. But it is not only members of minority groups who suffer the consequence of lack of preventive care. For example, obese adults are at risk for various serious conditions, including colorectal cancer. In all these conditions disease prevention and health promotion can increase longevity and decrease suffering and disability.

Prevention is very deceptive, however. At the heart of the problem is an overall misconception about how to motivate people to change their behavior. The accepted approach grows from the assumption, grounded in the health belief model, that if given the correct information, people will make the right decision. This misconception is reinforced by excessive reliance on the biomedical explanation of human nature. Individuals' perceptions, what sociologists call the "definition of the situation," are based on cultural norms and values and are reinforced by degree of autonomy and extent of social relationships; as a result, most formulas for lifestyle interventions are flawed. If you need proof, look at the results of abstinence-only and obesity-reduction education programs in our schools.

On the knowledge level, most people are not aware of the subtle but important differences between primary, secondary, and tertiary prevention. To be effective, prevention must work on all three levels. For my purposes, these levels can be divided into two groups: actions that can be taken at the societal and community level and those that can be part of the doctor-patient relationship. When it comes to primary prevention, to mention the obvious efforts, smoking cessation, nutritional counseling, and exercise regimens can be initiated in schools, churches, and voluntary organizations. Initiating them, however, is one thing; making them work is another. You can take the junk food machines out of the school cafeteria, but the kids can still get their burgers, fries, and pizza during their lunch break or after school. As I've said, lecturing does not work. An effective program will take a concerted effort both nationally and at the community level. It may even require some legislation, similar to that of the transfat ban in Manhattan's restaurants. In any case, the interventions must be based on a carefully designed plan, public support, and community cooperation. Regarding this last, a sincere attempt to understand how people perceive themselves in terms of their social situation can open the way to trust, growing from consideration. Purveyors of health promotion and disease prevention will need to design, establish, implement, and evaluate programs that detect and treat health risks early, preventing them from becoming life-threatening diseases.

Integrating prevention as a vital component of diagnosis and treatment in the doctor-patient relationship must be mandatory if this approach is to be successful. Both primary care and specialist doctors need to make prevention part of their practice. It can't be perfunctory, but must be done with follow-up that the patient recognizes and responds to. Practitioners need to understand and believe in the merits of prevention. Both the method and the philosophy can be cultivated throughout medical training. The office of the primary care physician is the ideal place for focusing on risk factors, especially for chronic diseases. The specialist, through the nature of his or her intervention, has the opportunity to promote prevention that plays a significant part in recovery after surgery or other invasive procedures.

Practitioners

As Ed O'Neil (2007) has observed, "Build[ing] more training facilities and enlarging class size" are not the solution. He goes on: "If the concentration of physicians makes for better health care it doesn't seem to be captured in the literature." The Institute of Medicine has put a great deal of effort into returning medicine to its professional roots. As I have stated repeatedly, I share their conviction that substantive reform in the organization and practice of medicine cannot take place without changing the way we train future doctors. It should also be clear by now that I feel strongly that being taught professionalism didactically is not the same as learning humanistic health care through experiential voluntary service.

To go back to the main theme of this book, RCSIP-type experiences not only lay the foundation for cultivating idealism in the student physician, but also prepare the future doctor for developing a humane relationship with patients. By now it should be apparent that I believe that to understand a patient more fully requires an awareness of the particular cultural milieu the patient comes from. Sensitivity to that person's culture and social status gives the practitioner a feeling for the obstacles faced by the patient. The need for cultural sensitivity, along with an awareness of the social and economic determinants of disease and illness, will be even more important with a potential future flood of previously uninsured people seeking health care, many of them from ethnic minority groups. Furthermore, our increasingly diversified society must be represented in the health and caring field. As I have mentioned previously, it is indefensible that so little effort by too many medical schools has been put into the recruitment and retention of students from underrepresented minority populations. Fortunately, the gender divide is gone, but the current situation reinforces a cultural and class divide.

It has been my experience over the past thirty-five years that most young men and women seeking a career in medicine do so for the right reasons, outlined throughout this book. Moreover, I am not discounting the continuing array of advances in medical education, such as, to mention only the most obvious, problem-based learning, preceptorships beginning in the first year, and fewer lectures. Clearly, every effort must be made to keep abreast of the exploding knowledge in medical research and clinical technique. My argument is, simply, that the core values—what many key figures in medicine called *professionalism*—have been pushed further and further from the heart of what makes for a compassionate and humanistic doctor. The very fact that the students who participate in RCSIP do so on their own gives credence to my explanation.

It is unrealistic to assume that major curricular reform can be instituted without difficulty. A great source of insight for me in this regard comes from the French sociologist Pierre Bourdieu (Swartz 1997). In his reflective sociology, he focuses on the synergy between culture and power as a basis for understanding highly organized structures such as academic health centers, which clearly qualify as representing a "stratified social system of hierarchy and domination that persists and reproduces intergenerationally without powerful resistance and without the conscious recognition of its members" (6). In our modern materialistic culture with its uncertainty and inconsistencies, value conflicts between being flexible and being affiliated are common. Contemporary medicine is a cauldron of such ambivalence. There is a myth about the freedom of being a doctor that dissolves quickly in the indoctrination system, unconsciously replaced by finding where you belong. Humanism takes a beating in the process.

Fundamentally, under these conditions medical education is incapable of reforming itself from the inside (for example, emphasizing professionalism) without a major overhaul. The primary stakeholders at the top—deans, department heads, highly regarded specialists—are too deeply entrenched in the traditional norms to allow changes that will affect their positions of power and control. RCSIP provided a venue in which students are able to wrest power and control from the administration and resist being completely socialized into this hierarchy, including fending off the not-so-subtle aspects circulated by "inside dopesters" (the purveyors of Hafferty's hidden curriculum). In other words, they are allowed to grow in clinical competence without losing their moral convictions.

Critical to the vitality of RCSIP and the broadening of the collective conscience of medicine is the constant wellspring of fresh, bright, inventive minds that each new class brings to the program. From a strictly learning-and-development perspective, RCSIP-type programs can be elevated to a well-defined and recognized position within the medical school system. This makes the program more significant than an extracurricular exercise would be, but in the process the program must not lose its autonomy. The students run their programs as a section head runs his or hers. This translational action lays the groundwork for a thorough curricular reform.

I would thus be remiss if I didn't try to show, even in the most rudimentary way, how these attributes and actions can be integrated into a more encompassing framework—an ideal curriculum—without contaminating an activity that, through its continual self-invention, has kept the voluntary service ethic alive. The curricular model that follows is generalized and can be adapted to the specific aims of any medical school. I'll even go so far as to say that the principles shown here are applicable to training in other professions, such as law, business, and education. A sensitivity to such virtues as idealism and humanism should resonate with us all.

Curricular Innovation

With support from the *inside*—dean, faculty committees, and student representatives—a new didactic *track* can be created independent of and complimentary to the community service experience. From the *outside,* pressure can be exerted by major medical organizations such as the Association of American Medical Colleges and the Institute of Medicine based on evidence from pilot programs, health policy reports, and health services research as well as public concern.

Nonetheless, it must be made clear that this new component of medical education is considered as important as the basic sciences, pathophysiology, and clinical medicine. Without such recognition the innovation is doomed from the start.

The responsibility for designing, implementing, and assessing this component would reside with the departments of social and preventive medicine, medical humanities, or similar sections that can or should be found in almost all medical schools. Representatives from both basic and clinical departments must be involved and committed to the track's success.

In appendix D, I present an initial format showing what such a curricular innovation might consist of. In addition, I propose a rationale of how to keep the community service component voluntary and at the same time fit it into the new curricular scheme. For the didactic component, a series of lecture topics from the humanities, social sciences, and public health can be developed. They should be few in number (for example, six one-hour lectures quarterly), but focused and relevant to the education of the humanistic physician. Small-group discussion (two two-hour sessions per quarter) would add an interactive dimension. During the clinical phase two grand rounds per core clerkship would suffice. This component must be substantive and carefully integrated. Emphasis must be placed on how the grand rounds fit into the biomedical components.

A special feature of the curricular innovation would offer students who are not interested in community service per se an opportunity to become engaged in some form of population research. The student who chooses epidemiology, for example, can investigate relevant social factors in clinical trials and longitudinal population studies. Just as interested medical students engage in various forms of bench research throughout their medical school training, the epidemiological experience would be important in seeing how data can be used as a basis for instituting policy.

Evaluation of the track as a pedagogical tool can be done through a pretest administered at matriculation and a posttest at graduation. Such assessments have the potential of being included as part of the licensing examinations.

The survey instruments used to collect these data must be well designed and carefully administered. A longitudinal schema must be created so that graduates can be followed throughout their careers.

In sum, I am proposing a social, community, and humanistic track that will add a needed dimension to the education of future physicians. Combined with voluntary community service, I believe, this approach will breed the humanism that is so desperately needed if medicine is to meet its social responsibility. Such a learning environment can play an important role in getting medicine reconnected to society by addressing issues pertinent to the welfare of us all.

Clearly, the problems and consequences of the proposed innovation are enormous. At best, what I am suggesting is only the beginning of merely thinking about how to proceed. The real test, of course, is to demonstrate that students who participate are clinically competent, ethically concerned, and socially conscious and are committed to being change agents at a time when reform in medicine is urgently needed.

After all is said and done, we cannot lose sight of the need to break the cycle of traditional medical education. A new *continuum* is required that incorporates humanistic values in the admissions process at the start and the moral order of residency programs at graduation. A full spectrum of humanistic values is the cultural basis of this learning and development activity. The students' idealism is primary in the selection process and nurtured throughout medical school. Graduate medical training fosters the same attitudes and beliefs. As the sequence evolves, a new and humane health care system can be created based on clinical competence, rigorous research, but, most fundamentally, social justice and equity.

Chapter 10

A Personal Reflection

The Staying Power of the Call of Service

Two Kinds of Intelligence

There are two kinds of intelligence: one,
    required
as a child in school, memorizes facts and
    concepts
from the books and what the teacher says,
collecting information from the traditional
    sciences
as well as from the new sciences.
With such intelligence you rise in the
    world.
You get ranked ahead or behind others
in regards to your competence in retaining
information. You stroll with this
    intelligence
in and out of fields of knowledge, getting
    always more
marks on your preserving tablets.
There is another kind of tablet, one
already completed and preserved inside
    you.
A spring overflowing its springbox.
    A freshness

in the center of the chest. This other
  intelligence
does not turn yellow or stagnate. It's fluid,
and it doesn't move from outside to inside
through conduits of plumbing-learning.
This second knowing is a fountainhead
from within you, moving out.

—Rumi, thirteenth-century Persian poet, "Two
Kinds of Intelligence"

Vancouver 2000

In March 2000, I was asked to make a presentation on "humanitarianism" at the Ninth International Health in Medical Education Conference in Vancouver, British Columbia. My session was one of four scheduled for this time slot, after lunch on the second day of the conference. Much to my surprise, the room was packed, primarily with medical students from across the United States and Canada. Although I had prepared some material based on my involvement with the Health of the Public program and my discussions with Fred Hafferty on the culture of medical education, I knew my best way of engaging this very eager-looking group was to begin by asking them some basic questions. I must say it was one of the most exciting sessions I'd had with a group of students in such a setting for a long time.

I started by asking why this particular session (Towards a Humanitarian Cause) interested them. They were not inhibited! The responses came from a variety of directions, but the central theme, as far as they were concerned, was that "traditional medical education" was not interested in, let alone committed to, providing a learning environment that encouraged humanitarianism. As the discussion increased in intensity, the students started using the term *compassion* more than *humanitarianism*. When I asked why, one of the students said *humanitarianism* sounded phony: it was the kind of word that rich people used to show that they wanted to help less fortunate people by giving large donations to some favorite charity or institution. Many students nodded their agreement. Another raised the term *altruism,* saying it meant "giving freely of yourself." Wasn't that compassion? I asked. Yes, but wasn't altruism giving of one's self to people who really needed it? Another said there was no personal reward (money or status) when you take care of the poor.

Next I asked why they were interested in international health. Again I was greeted with a barrage of answers. The majority of students stressed that they did not want to be "cultural tourists," spending a few weeks or a month in some exotic place to get a little flavor of what it was like but unwilling to do more than that. For those in the room, international health meant placing themselves in a different culture, primarily a developing country, not only to learn about the people and the hardships they face but also to help in any way they could, and that meant not necessarily clinically. I also got the feeling that going abroad was seen as a way of "breaking out" from a kind of insularity that students felt was created by the rigidity of medical education in the academic health center. When medical school started to "eat them up," they needed to get as far away as possible. A corollary focus was a quest for a global perspective. What I heard most often in this discussion was that the only way to truly understand multiculturalism in our society was to go to the roots of that particular culture (by going to, for example, South Africa or Guatemala). On further probing, I sensed that they saw themselves as future doctors with a view that took in the world, rather than as being purely North American.

The discussion got really hot when I raised the issue of professionalism. Comments were quite varied and loaded with passion and anger. There were some students, probably the most outspoken and radical, who rejected the concept without hesitation. For them, *professional* meant a rigid set of standards that allowed the physician to remain "above" the patient. I asked them what trait best described what they meant. One of the more outspoken replied, "Authority." Another group of students leery of viewing medicine as a profession saw their motivation to become doctors as a "calling" in the spiritual sense. I saw a spirit reminiscent of Saint Anthony's in their unencumbered faith that becoming a doctor was, in the most simple and humble fashion, a way of loving people by caring for them. There was no mention of autonomy, standards, screening, or any of the other aspects of professionalism that are fundamental to contemporary American medicine's attempts to redefine itself.

When I asked, as a follow-up question, if they were getting a professional education, I thought (at least in retrospect) I heard a collective bitter, cynical laugh. For this group of students—activists, international health participants, advocates for the indigent and disenfranchised—professionalism stood for an elitism that in essence was a barrier to their idealism as the basis for wanting to become a physician in the first place. Their message was essentially the same as that of the RCSIP participants—to be humane you must understand the humanity of others. This may seem obvious, but it is in fact elusive and deceptive.

Chicago 2000

Upon returning to Chicago, my head still spinning, I discussed all this with Claudia, my partner in coordinating our community service projects. Although the focus was on international health, the Vancouver experience had strong implications for everything we were trying to accomplish and reinforced my motivation to describe and explain what we had observed among our student participants over the past decade. It was the inspiration I needed to write this book.

During the course of documenting the long, illustrious history of these service activities, I was able, on looking back, to put to rest one of my initial fears: what Max Weber referred to as the "routinization of charisma" (Gerth and Mills 1958, 54). Weber was the first to use the concept of charisma—in the original Greek meaning of "touched by God"—to describe leaders of exceptional magnetism who not only drew people to them but also eventually got those people to become devoted followers in a state of euphoria and excitement over something new and different. He also wrote extensively about bureaucracy, which he characterized as an "iron cage." For Weber routinization took place when the excitement had waned and the process had become more routine, usually in the form of a bureaucracy. My concern was that once the RCSIP projects were operating smoothly, they would become routine and the passion and enthusiasm that made the programs so exhilarating would wane. This has not been the case. Contrary to my fears, RCSIP continues to grow and evolve.

Phase 2

I have recently tried to update the status of RCSIP. I will call this period (2000–2007) the start of phase 2. The logical way of going about this is to see which of the original programs are continuing, which ones no longer exist, and which ones are new. Three of the four initial clinics continue to provide health care to the uninsured, members of disadvantaged minority groups, and the homeless.

RCSIP doctors and students volunteer one evening a week at CommunityHealth, still the exception among free clinics because of its full laboratory, pharmacy, and range of services, from routine physicals and immunizations to complicated diagnoses and treatment modalities. For example, Dr. Paul Jones, an otolaryngologist who for a time was director of RCSIP, offers his specialty services one day each month.

The Pilsen clinic serving the homeless has become an accepted and recognized community institution and, in the process, has broadened its patient base to include women and children. This free clinic is the predominant source of health care for recent Mexican immigrants. Dr. Maria Brown remains the people's doctor and continues to be the mentor to and model for many idealistic students. In 2005 she was selected as a member of the prestigious Mark Lepper Society, which is composed of distinguished teachers.

The clinic at the Franciscan House of Mary and Joseph homeless shelter, one of the original clinics started by RCSIP, has become a permanent part of their services. Like the clinic at Pilsen, it is a major source of medical care for many of the shelter's residents. Dr. Steve Rothschild, one of the most committed of the original physicians to collaborate with the students, now oversees the provision of medical services. Dr. Stephanie Luther, a former student activist and now a Rush faculty member, is Dr. Rothschild's partner in supervising the students.

Rush students and physicians no longer participate at St. Basil's, although there is a possibility that the relationship can be reactivated. From the St. Basil's side, doctors and students from the University of Chicago and other Chicago medical schools provide services. From the Rush side the number of clinical experiences continues to expand, so RCSIP members are not desperately seeking new sites.

Mobile community health care services are offered through two vans. The Mammovan, which began operating in the late 1990s, is a mobile mammography station that travels within Cook County providing free mammograms to underserved women. The institutional home of the van is the Fantus Clinic of the John H. Stroger Hospital (formerly Cook County Hospital), where the students also assist in taking mammograms. The Medical Outreach Van gives the students a chance to work with underserved people directly on the streets of Chicago. One aspect of the program, called Open Door and overseen by Dr. Brown, is to go to Lower Wacker Drive (the only street remaining from the devastating Chicago Fire), which, because it is covered, has become a gathering place for the homeless and former or active drug users. A large group of "residents" huddle together there during Chicago's deep-freeze winters.

Another new RCSIP involvement is the Kids Shelter Improvement Project. In 2005 it was estimated that more than twenty-six thousand children and adolescents are homeless in Illinois over the course of a year. They lack basic primary care and many do not receive routine childhood immunizations. This free health care service is a collaborative effort involving students and faculty from Rush and the University of Chicago and residents from Stroger Hospital. Kids Shelter is an outreach program: teams of doctors and students travel to more than a dozen homeless shelters to administer on-site medical services.

What used to be called One Shot Deals has evolved into RU Caring. In the new program, students from medicine, nursing, occupational therapy, nutrition, audiology, health systems management, and clinical laboratory sciences join forces to offer a full spectrum of health-related events at local schools. The services offered are broad and bold in execution. Besides some hands-on clinical efforts such as immunizations, other health-related programs consist of a project to confront obesity as well as to emphasize health and fitness. An example of this group's readiness to help was their collection of a truckload of hygiene products from Rush departments and sections that were distributed to Katrina survivors who were relocated in Chicago.

Of particular interest are the school-based health centers operated by the College of Nursing at Crane and Orr High Schools, close to Rush on the Near West Side. In offering comprehensive medical care and behavioral counseling, the centers seek to keep adolescents healthy, in school, and functioning well emotionally. In these settings the nursing students supervise the medical students, but through respect and cooperation, they work as a team.

Since the Chicago public schools have established their own safe-sex and AIDS-prevention curriculum, there is no longer a need for RAIDS. Cyrus the Virus has graduated and is a practicing psychiatrist in San Francisco, helping children who are recent arrivals from countries where war and torture are common and who are suffering from posttraumatic stress disorder. But the Pediatric AIDS Support Program is alive and fully operating as a well-integrated part of the Infectious Disease Department AIDS program, which still is directed by Dr. Ram Yogev, at Children's Memorial Hospital on Chicago's North Side. In 2005, twenty-three kids were "adopted" by Rush students.

Casa Guatemala remains a stable community center in a poor transient area, serving immigrants, some of them political refugees, from Central and South America. Because of students' earlier work, the staff is able to teach the new arrivals how to use the existing government health system. Many of the residents of Uptown still use CommunityHealth as a source of medical service.

Over the past five years or more, the Chicago Housing Authority has slowly dismantled Henry Horner Homes. The era of the high-rise housing project is over in Chicago, and in its place are new low-rise units not concentrated in one particular community. The majority of families from Horner have moved to other neighborhoods. Nonetheless, the reconstruction and relocation process will take a long time and is dependent on federal government funding.

The nonclinical programs, which offer a variety of services that are not strictly medical, have continued to proliferate over the past five years. The Henry Horner Tutoring Program, one of the originals, is still going in the Major

Adams Academy, the former Boys and Girls Club. The medical students help kids with math and English and give them tips on how to organize time for doing their homework.

Casa Juan Diego Tutoring is modeled after the Horner program. It is located in the youth center sponsored by St. Pius Catholic Church at the edge of the Pilsen neighborhood. Besides the usual tutoring and homework activities, the medical students perform interactive, hands-on science experiments that have become a big hit with children.

Mariah's Place is a shelter for homeless women that is affiliated with Deborah's Place, the largest supplier of support housing for homeless women in Chicago. Their aim is to end the cycle of homelessness by helping women to move out of their current situation and start a new life. At Mariah's Place, Rush students become mentors and advocates for the women, many of whom suffer from the physical and psychological effects of abuse. The medical students, under the guidance of a faculty mentor, give breast and pelvic examinations. They also provide valuable health and wellness information regarding diabetes, hypertension, and the signs of mental illness. The students are not only astute in their knowledge but also sensitive in how they present the information. Again, the key to success is establishing relationships based on openness, trust, and acceptance.

Other educational and advisory projects include community education and outreach done in conjunction with the Salvation Army Temple located at a fifteen-minute walk from Rush. The children and teenagers especially enjoy tours of the medical center. The health educators, following the precedent set by RAIDS, visit elementary and middle schools within the medical-center region to promote health as a way of preventing disease. The "curriculum" is based on such topics as sexual and reproductive health, nutrition, hygiene, and puberty. An interesting spin-off from what was formerly called Youth Link is VD Ed in which RCSIP participants volunteer in the Stroger Hospital emergency room, where they approach adolescents about sexual issues including HIV, sexually transmitted diseases, and unwanted pregnancies. The medical students are very sensitive and take care to avoid being preachy and making moral judgments. The emergency room doctors support the students and encourage the teenagers to listen to their message.

There are also a number of programs that are based on the same premise of following or "adopting" one person that was used in the creation of the Big Sib program for children with AIDS. The Buddies program matches the medical students with chronically ill children. This is not a medical care program; the main focus is friendship and support. At the Bowman Geriatric Center, located at Rush, students spend time with elderly residents, listening, reading, taking walks, and basically being a friend. In the Maternal Advocates Program, a RCSIP member is paired with an expectant teen mother from the Rush-Advocate Health and Family Clinic, which is also housed in the medical center. As in the prenatal clinic at St. Basil's, the student advocate serves as a source of support throughout a woman's pregnancy and, in some cases, after the delivery.

Besides the continuation of old programs and the addition of new ones, a number of other developments have emerged. First, RCSIP is recognized as a permanent component of the medical school and is funded by the Rush University Medical Center. Second, based on mechanisms created during the 1990s, the current system is well structured and organized. Third, data collection has been built into the new operation, including questions about awareness of RCSIP as a factor in applying to Rush and a protocol for following participants after graduation. Since 2000, survey data has shown that more than 80 percent of medical college matriculants were aware of RCSIP when they applied for admission. More than one-third stated that it was a major factor in deciding to come to Rush. Another 50 percent said it played some role in their decision. Finally, I want to point out that the new director, Sharon Gates, is much loved and admired by the students. She is keeping a tradition alive that Claudia and I both cherish.

A group of current RCSIP participants emphatically confirm that the major difference between learning in RCSIP and in preceptorships is that the former allows them to feel free and collegial with their mentor whereas the latter is stressful and competitive because they are graded. It is fair to say that RCSIP continues to evolve, expand, and adapt to the times. I have solicited a few narratives from current medical student participants to find out what RCSIP means to them personally, and a sample of their statements follows.

This is what Monica Mazda, a second-year student, has to say:

> My experiences in RCSIP have been the most rewarding experiences I have had in medical school so far. Volunteer work has been a very important part of my life ever since high school, but the stresses of medical school [made it seem] like it would be hard to continue volunteering. . . . I found myself feeling quite empty when I have not done anything for others for some time, and spending two years being completely selfish with my time I'm afraid would make me quite miserable.
>
> RCSIP is so well organized that it also makes it a lot easier to volunteer. . . . I have been able to enjoy tutoring students at Henry Horner, steering at CHC [CommunityHealth Clinic], and volunteering with Franciscan, Mobile Van, and RU Caring. Horner is a wonderful

experience. . . . It is very fulfilling whenever one of them really seems to understand what you have taught them. But when the fourth-grade girl I was tutoring could not write the alphabet, I also started realizing how different the lives of these children are than where I grew up.

Medical school has been extremely hard for me and being at [CHC] in charge of my peers and answering questions for the attendings has on several occasions brought my confidence back.

I think RCSIP and Sharon are two big reasons that Rush students are the happiest med students in Chicago.

Jessica Sinnott, also a second-year student, said this:

My involvement in RCSIP programs has been a tremendous addition to my education at Rush.

When deciding to come to Rush, I was excited about the possibility of being involved with clinics, but I had no idea how much of an impact the experience would have on me. [At] Pilsen I have really enjoyed getting to know a bit about the homeless "network" in Chicago—meaning where and how people go to get what they need regarding health care, food, shelter, and the like. I am hoping to continue working with an underserved population once I am done with my training.

I have also worked closely with the Door of Hope project, which is more on-the-street kind of service, and it has been neat to have some continuity with the people staying there, getting to know their stories and building relationships. From an educational standpoint, RCSIP programs have been invaluable. [Dr. Brown] has been an excellent mentor by being willing to answer questions, help write notes, and explain disease. She brings a lot of knowledge about the underserved population to us and has helped me understand many things—from how to administer a PPD [a purified protein derivative injected in the skin to test for tuberculosis] to how to appropriately interview about substance abuse. . . . To work closely with patients and ask questions in a relaxed environment has helped me build confidence. . . .

I consider myself blessed for having had the chance to be involved with RCSIP, both for its educational and personal value.

My Personal Reflection

When I look at my RCSIP experiences, my greatest source of enlightenment, as well as satisfaction, was the students, especially the activists whom I have personally observed for more than a decade. These students were so-called

Generation Xers, the children of baby boomers who came into an untrusting, self-centered world.[1] The reason they found participating in these community service activities so satisfying was that it filled a gap and provided something that was missing not only from their formal education, but also from their sense of purpose in life. Many of them didn't even know what was missing until they got outside the medical school and into settings that actually required them to work together, where they didn't have to compete with one another. Through common tasks and shared goals, they learned the efficacy of Putnam's (2000) idea of social capital, that is, those intangibles—goodwill, fellowship, social intercourse—that count for most in the daily lives of people. In the process, they also learned about the health and social needs of the poor and disadvantaged patient or client as well as about the communities where they volunteered. Their personal reflections on these issues constituted the main theme of the numerous discussions Claudia and I had with them individually or in small groups.

By observing students, talking with them, and reflecting with them, I have learned that much of the ambivalence they feel toward the system under which they are trained comes from two factors: such a system thwarts their idealism by constraining their ability to act according to their values, and the profession is remiss when it come to keeping its social contract with society. The narratives by the students and the doctors are especially illuminating about their emotional side. Their emotions involved judgments about what they believed was important not exclusively for a doctor but essentially for a human being. In this regard, they felt free to express their feelings openly. The emotions they experienced were the psychological fuel that fired their idealism.

In a sociopolitical vein, what community service and international health participation have in common is the audacity of attempting to lay the foundation for a just and equitable world. More now than ever, as Geoffrey Rose (1993) has observed, "medicine and politics are irrevocably intertwined." By their very action, participants are making a statement and taking a stance. Social action is a salient component of RCSIP, and to overlook its significance to what the program was trying to achieve is to turn one's back on reality. Besides its intrinsic worth, RCSIP, by channeling the idealism the students bring to medical school through voluntary services that are humanistic and pragmatic, is a change agent for reconnecting medicine to society.

The students taught me a lot. They showed me that personal satisfaction and social responsibility are not at odds. When it comes to Rush medical students, this much I know for sure: the hard-core students who participated in RCSIP saw themselves as advocates for the underserved. Furthermore, they saw the services they provided, whether lowering blood pressure or being a buddy to a kid with congenital heart disease, as both personal and social acts. Through the very act of looking after the well-being of those under their care, they become personally responsible for each one. Taking care of people in an economically deprived community fosters social responsibility. In other words, it soon becomes apparent that if you are going to keep your patients or clients healthy, something must be done to treat the community or social environment that was instrumental in creating the negative situation. This awareness, this wisdom, this confrontation with oppressive conditions does not come from textbooks, interesting presentations in the lecture hall, or carefully developed case studies; it comes from being absorbed into the social reality of what constitutes humanity.

Reading Paul Farmer's *Pathologies of Power* (2003) gave me further insight. Since Farmer is committed to entire country populations (the people of Haiti, prisoners in Russia) whose poverty and deprivation are a way of life, he represents the ideal. It's not that I hadn't thought about social injustice and violations of human rights (what he calls a "structure of violence") that is always at stake for those whom Frantz Fanon named "the wretched of the earth." Farmer's ability to confront these dreadful and inhumane conditions and their accompanying diseases (tuberculosis, AIDS) with such passion and anger, wisdom and experience, makes his the approach to emulate. But we can't all go to the Haitis of the world (regardless of how great the need). What we can do at home, in the richest country on the face of the earth, is to reach out to those who are outside the system, to train future health professionals by exposing them to these conditions, and, without reservation, become politically active through organizations such as Physicians for Social Responsibility, establishing new social movements, or even working from within the current system to fight for the real changes that are needed.

In short, it is the "vision thing." Not only will the physicians with RCSIP-type experience practice a more humanistic and socially responsible medicine, but they also will bring a new vision for cultivating the seeds of reform. They are aware that health and disease are not only biophysical entities but also socio-cultural and environmental phenomena. They are the future section heads, department chairs, center directors, and medical school deans. The vision they bring is needed for influencing health policy that directly addresses the political and social implications of promoting health for all.

Sources of Funding for RCSIP

Funding Source	Amount
The AT&T Corporation	$50,000
1991–1993	
The Lloyd A. Fry Foundation	300,000
1991–1995	
The Health of the Public Group	300,000
Sponsored by the Robert Wood Johnson Foundation, the PEW Charitable Trust, in conjunction with the Rockefeller Foundation	
1993–1997	
The Northern Trust Company	240,000
1993–1999; 1999–2005	
Illinois Department of Public Health	88,500
Office of Women's Health	
1998–1999; 2000–2002	
Today's Chicago Women	20,000
1999–2000	
Illinois Violence Prevention Authority	70,000
1999–2001	
Polk Brothers Foundation	140,000
1999–2002	
Department of Health and Human Services	476,000
Bureau of Primary Health Care	
1999–2003	
Total	$1,684,500

Guidelines for Maintaining Safety and Security

Unfortunately, we live in a society where violent acts are not uncommon. No community or person is immune, regardless of their power, position, or sophisticated security system. Statistics also show that certain areas are pockets of crime and violence. This is a fact. So, what does this mean? Never leave the protective environment (which itself is no guarantee) of your home, neighborhood, or academic center? Of course not! Many people spend the majority of their lives in these communities. They are law-abiding citizens; family members; and decent, loving human beings. They have opened their neighborhoods, homes, and hearts to many of us.

Chicago is a fantastic city—one of the most culturally diverse in the world. The only way to see and know the city is to experience it personally. That is what this program is all about. The only real way to learn about the health of the public is to go where the public is—in the community. By taking the following simple precautions, you should be able to participate fully in these activities, which we think you will find not only edifying but also fun:

- Travel in groups, two or more per vehicle, and keep the doors locked and windows closed.
- Do not wear expensive clothes, jewelry, or things that make you an inviting target.
- Don't go down any side streets or dead ends unless you are familiar with the main streets. Know your way in and out of the community.
- Don't leave *anything* in the car. If you have a cell phone, lock it up along with other enticing possessions before you leave. If someone sees you putting things in your trunk after you have parked, they may break a window to get in.
- When going to a particular site (a health clinic, a school), park in designated areas or as close to the site as possible.
- Whenever you go on foot, go in groups. No exceptions—the loner is the most vulnerable.
- Avoid dark and isolated places. At a clinic, you want to be identified as someone who is giving voluntary service there.
- Stay away from any groups hanging out on street corners, in front of liquor stores, and the like. Never imitate hand signals or other movements.

- Don't go near any place or approach anyone if you feel the least bit uncomfortable.
- Be cool; be savvy; and don't, under any condition, take any unnecessary risks.
- Be respectful at all times.
- Finally, remember that students in RCSIP have been going to inner-city communities and neighborhoods (frequently at night) since 1990. By following these simple precautions they have remained safe, secure, and happy. In fact, they are loved and respected in most of the places where they volunteer.

Publications and Presentations of RCSIP Participants

P. DeGolia, E. Thompson, J. England, and E. Eckenfels, "The Rush Primary Care Clinics Project: A Student-Generated Model for Health Promotion and Disease Prevention through Education and Practice in a Medically Underserved Community." *Proceeding of the 1990 Conference of Community Responsive Practice,* March 1990.

E. Eckenfels, J. May, and G. Barley, "Student-Generated Community-Oriented Projects: Personal Learning and Development through Community Service." *Academic Medicine* 65, no. 9, Supplement, September 1990.

E. Eckenfels, C. Baier, J. Billings, and M. Bardack, "Community Service Initiatives as a Source of Student Learning and Development in Medical School." *Proceedings of the Group on Educational Affairs,* AAMC, November 1991.

E. Eckenfels, D. Self, D. Baldwin, and C. Baier, "Three Perspectives for Enhancing Medical Students' Values and Beliefs to Become Humane and Culturally Sensitive Physicians." *Academic Medicine* 67, no. 10, Supplement, 1992.

E. Eckenfels, "The Rush Community Service Initiatives Program: A Model to Enhance Community Health through Student-Faculty Collaboration." Annual Meeting of the AAHC, September 1992.

M. Bardack, S. Thompson, and E. Eckenfels, "The Rush Prenatal Program at St. Basil's Free People's Clinic: Personal Learning and Development through Active Community Service." AAMC Annual Meeting, OSR presentations, November 1992.

K. Zorek and C. Baier, "Rush Students Organize Health-Care Symposium" *The Physician* 41, 1992.

M. Bardack and S. Thompson, Secretary for Health and Human Services' Award for Innovations in Health Promotion and Disease Prevention, 1992.

E. Eckenfels, "The Rush Community Service Initiatives Program: A Model to Enhance Community Health through Student-Faculty Collaboration." In W. D. Skelton and M. Osterweis, eds., *Promoting Community Health: The Role of the Academic Health Center.* Washington, DC: Association of Academic Health Centers, 1993.

M. Bardack and S. Thompson, "Model Prenatal Program of Rush Medical College at St. Basil's Free People's Clinic." *Public Health Reports* 105, no. 2, 1993.

E. Eckenfels, "U.S. Experiences with Community Service: The Urban Chicago Perspective." Pan American Health Organization Conference, March, 1993.

E. Eckenfels, "Health Services in the Schools: Problems and Solutions." Institute of Medicine Conference, May 1993.

C. Baier, S. Crandall, J. Gotlieb, and E. Eckenfels, "Community-Based Education and Service Strategies in Medical Education: Revitalizing Curricula to Prevent Burnout and Promote Authentic Development among Medical Students." Paper presented at the annual meeting of the Association of American Medical Colleges, November 1993.

S. Baman, D. Graham, and C. Baier, "The Student Coalition for Community Service." AAMC Annual Meetings, OSR Presentation, November 1993.

S. Lustig, Secretary of Health and Human Services' Award for Innovations in Health Promotion and Disease Prevention, 1993.

S. Lustig, C. Baier, S. Daugherty, and E. Eckenfels, "Preventing the Tragic with Magic: The AIDS Prevention Magic Show." International Conference on AIDS Education, November 1993.

E. Eckenfels, "The Practice of Medicine: Prognosis for the Future." Symposium sponsored by the Student Coalition for Community Service and AMSA's General Physicians in Training, January 1994.

M. Bardack, C. Baier, and E. Eckenfels, "Patients' Perceptions of Quality of Care and Students' Assessment of Learning and Development of a Student-Run Prenatal Clinic." *Proceedings of Prevention '94,* March 1994.

E. Eckenfels, "Community Service in Medical Education." OSR Regional Meeting, April 1994.

S. Lustig, "Preventing the Tragic with Magic: The AIDS Prevention Magic Show." *Public Health Reports* 109, no. 2, 1994.

E. Eckenfels, C. Baier, K. Turner-Roan, and A. Sanchez, "Enhancing the Learning and Development of Medical Students through Community Service." In *Effective Learning—Effective Teaching—Effective Service: Voices from the Field on Improving Education through Community Service-Learning.* Youth Service America's Working Group on National and Community Service Policy, Washington, DC, 1994.

C. Baier, "Integrating Community Awareness and Service within a Traditional Medical Education Experience: The Rush Community Service Initiatives Program." *Annals of Behavioral Science in Medical Education* 1, no. 1:52–53, 1994.

K. Turner-Roan, "Is Asthma Affecting More Inner-City Kids Than We Realized?" *People Wise* 2, no. 1, 1994.

T. Palmer, E. Eckenfels, C. Baier, and K. Turner-Roan, "The Rush Community Service Initiatives Program." Poster, Thirteenth Annual Northeast Regional Meeting of Teachers of Family Medicine, October 1994.

C. Baier and E. Eckenfels, "Student-Generated Community Service and Educational Programs: Preparing Future Physicians for Meeting Societal Needs in the Twenty-first Century." Paper presented at the Annual Meeting of the Association for Behavioral Sciencesin Medical Education October 1994.

E. Eckenfels, "In Search of Authentic Learning and Development among Medical Students: A Reassessment of the Role of the Social Sciences in Medical Education." *Proceedings of the Association for Behavioral Sciences in Medical Education Annual Meeting,* October 1994.

E. Eckenfels, C. Baier, and K. Turner-Roan, "The Rush Community Service Initiatives Program: A Health of the Public Participant." *Proceedings of the American Public Health Association Annual Meeting,* November 1994.

E. Eckenfels, "Community Service." Panelist, the Student Coalition for Community Service and AMSA's Generalist Physicians in Training Second Annual Symposium, January 1995.

C. Baier, "Indigenous Community Members as Health Care Providers: A Discussion." Poster, Health of the Public Annual Meeting, January 1995.

L. Francis, M. Earing, Y. Choi, and C. Baier, "Training Pre-clinical Medical Students to Do Functional Assessments: A Successful Community Partnership." American Association on Aging Annual Meeting, March 1995.

E. Eckenfels, "Public Health Services for Latinos in Chicago." Panel, University of Chicago II Symposium on Latin American Human Rights, April 1995.

M. Planta and S. Lustig, Recognizing Tomorrow's Leaders Today. AMA/Glaxo Achievement Award, Washington, D.C., April 1995.

C. Baier, K. Turner-Roan, G. Henry, J. Rockford, and T. Allen, "Rush Community Service Initiatives: The Henry Horner Pediatric Asthma Program." Pharmaceutical Representative Clinical Training Program for Allen & Hanburys/Glaxo, Chicago, May/October/November 1995.

C. Baier, G. Garfield, G. Mart, and K. Flannery, "The Franciscan Brothers Homeless Shelter Clinic." Panel, the Rush Alumni Executive Council, September 1995.

C. Baier, "Enhancing the Learning and Development of Medical Students through Community Service: A Model for Fostering Social Responsibility, Educational Reform, and Provider Collaboration." Roundtable, American Public Health Association Conference, November 1995.

S. Banman, M. Planta, and C. Baier, "Community Generated, Community Run: The Henry Horner Pediatric Asthma Program." Poster, American Medical Student Association National Multidisciplinary Conference on Healthy Communities, December 1995.

E. Eckenfels, C. Baier, C. Garfield, S. Powell, A. Price, A. Schaffner, and G. Carreon, "Learning through Service: The Rush Community Service Initiatives Program." Workshop, the Association of American Medical Colleges Central Group on Educational Affairs Annual Conference, April 1996.

E. Eckenfels, "Using Managed Care to Teach Students to Think Critically." Annual Meeting of the Association of Behavior Science in Medical Education, October 1996.

RCSIP as co-recipient with Children's Memorial Hospital of the Illinois Department of Public Health's third Annual World AIDS Day Award for Exceptional Merit to an organization for the Pediatric AIDS Big Sib program, November 1996.

D. Allen, "Working with Asthma in the Henry Horner Community." *Our Voices: Westhaven Community Newsletter* 4, December 1996.

G. Carron and M. Fernandez, "The Pediatric AIDS Big Sib Program." Presented at the Rush–Presbyterian–St. Luke's and Cook County Medical Centers World AIDS events, December 1996.

A. Bonesho, C. Hagedorn, R. Houlahan, and R. Schaefer, "The Rush Community Service Initiatives Program." Poster, American Medical Association/Chicago Medical Society Annual Conference, February 1997.

J. Tess, C. Baier, E. Eckenfels, and R. Yogev, "Medical Students Act as Big Brothers/Sisters to Support HIV-Infected Children's Psychosocial Needs." *Archives of Pediatric and Adolescent Medicine* 151, February 1997.

S. Baman, Recognizing Tomorrow's Leaders Today. AMA/Glaxo Achievement Award, Philadelphia, March 1997.

C. Baier, M. Adiga, G. Henry, and S. Green, "The Henry Horner Pediatric Asthma Program." Breakout session, International Medical Education Consortium Annual Conference, March 1997.

N. Sehgal, "Student Involvement at the CommunityHealth Free Clinic." Breakout session, International Health and Medical Educational Consortium Annual Conference, March 1997.

C. Baier, "Student-Generated Community Service and Education Programs." Primary Care for the Underserved, Fifth Annual Conference, May 1997.

L. Koch, A. Sivan, and C. Baier, "Refugee Youth at Risk: A Review of Issues Surrounding Youth and Gang Violence." American Public Health Association Annual Meeting, November 1997.

E. Eckenfels, "Contemporary Medical Students' Quest for Self-Fulfillment through Community Service." *Academic Medicine* 72, December 1997.

T. Palmer, C. Baier, S. Daugherty, and E. Eckenfels, "The Need for Longitudinal Evaluation for Community Service Programs." Family Medicine Research Forum, McNeal Hospital, Chicago, June 1998.

C. Baier, "Community-Based Asthma Education and Case Management: Reaching the Underserved." Children at Risk: Environmental Health Treats in the Great Lakes Region, EPA/ATSDR Regional Conference, July 1998.

M. Adiga, A. Sivan, C. Baier, and L. Koch, "Gang Prevention with Refugee Youth." Paper presented at the Twenty-fifth Annual Convention of the Association of Haitian Physicians Abroad, July 1998.

E. Eckenfels, "Innovation in Education and Service: The Rush Community Service Initiatives Program." International Conference on Health Service Programs and Institutions, Cuernavaca, Mexico, July 1998.

C. Baier, E. Eckenfels, and M. Adiga, "The Need for Longitudinal Evaluation of Community Service: Lessons Learned from the Rush Community Service Initiatives Program." Primary Care Education for the Twenty-first Century: Lessons from National Initiatives, September 1998.

E. Eckenfels and F. Hafferty, "An Assessment of the Medical School Objectives Program: Using Community Service to Enhance Students' Idealism and Altruism." American Association of Medical Colleges, November 1998.

C. Baier, T. Palmer, S. Daugherty, and E. Eckenfels, "The Need for Longitudinal Evaluation of Community Service Programs: Lessons Learned from the Rush Community Service Initiatives Program." Paper presented at the Annual Meeting of the American Association of Medical Colleges, November 1998.

E. Eckenfels, R. McKersie, and G. Maker, "Voluntary Community Service Programs: Medical Students' Initiatives to Reach the Community." American Association of Medical Colleges, November 1998.

E. Eckenfels, "The Balance between Research and Service: The Importance of Evaluating Community Service Program." Chicago Urban Schweitzer Fellowships Program Symposium, January 1999.

J. Mendoza, "The Buddies Community Service Program." American Medical Student Association National Conference, March 1999.

E. Grant, S. Daugherty, T. Li, E. Eckenfels, C. Baier, and K. Weiss, "Early Results of a Community Asthma Knowledge and Attitude Survey." ALA/ATS International Conference, April 1999.

C. Baier and G. Henry, "RCSIP's Henry Horner Pediatric Asthma Program." University of Illinois Great Cities Institute, International Center for Health Leadership Development, Partnership Luncheon Series, May 1999.

E. Eckenfels and W. Addington, "Student-Generated Initiatives for Community Service and International Health: The Vision of the Academic Health Center for the Third Millennium." Universities and the Health of the Disadvantaged: A Global Conference, Tucson, Arizona, August, 1999.

E. Eckenfels, F. Hafferty, and J. O'Donnell, "Making Future Physicians More Altruistic: Affirmation, Acquisition, and Evaluation." AAMC Annual Meeting, Washington, D.C., October, 1999.

E. Eckenfels, "Enhancing the Learning and Development of Contemporary Medical Students Through Community Service." Central American Conference on Public Health and Human Rights, Havana, Cuba, August 2000.

E. Eckenfels, "The Case for Keeping Community Service Voluntary: Narratives from the Rush Community Service Initiatives Program." In D. Wear and J. Bickel, eds., *Education for Professionalism: Creating a Culture of Humanism in Medical Education.* University of Iowa Press, Iowa City, 2000.

F. Hafferty and E. Eckenfels, "The Perils of Becoming an Altruistic Physician: The Me Generation Enters Medical School." Association of Behavioral Sciences in Medical Education Annual Meeting, Falmouth, MA, September 2001.

E. Eckenfels, "The Struggle for the Soul of Medicine." *Journal of ABSAME* 10, no. 1, Spring 2004.

The Social Medicine, Community Health, and Human Rights Curriculum

Has there been any change in the last 50 years?
Has there been none? Those of you in this room
should know. And, if so, what caused that
change to occur?

—Nicholas Christakis, *Interim Report of the Acadia
Institute on Undergraduate Medical Education*

Is it possible to integrate humanistic attributes and actions in a more encompassing framework—a new curriculum—without contaminating an activity that, through participants' enthusiasm, has kept the service ethic alive? There are two major dilemmas that restrict any proposed reforms based on RCSIP. First, how can programs be required and voluntary at the same time? Second, can medical school faculty who are deeply invested in the model of the traditional curriculum be persuaded to change without causing serious resentment? What I am proposing is, on the surface, both well-nigh impossible and extremely controversial.

My reference in what follows is Rush, but my model, if feasible, applies to American medical education in general. The very thought of an intellectual and experiential widening of the curriculum brings shivers down the spines of the basic scientists who hang on tenaciously to every course hour they feel they have won through bloody scrimmages with their clinical counterparts. The myth of the traditional curriculum as the only way to educate must be debunked slowly but firmly. What the "traditionalists" actually believe, without realizing it, is that the culture of medical education is unalterable. But culture is fluid, not static, and that means the culture of medical school can change, but it will take serious effort by those committed to reform.

When I have cautiously raised the idea of integrating our voluntary service programs into the existing curriculum, a typical response has been "The dean has the power to do it, and, if he or she says so, it will happen." I presume that this notion is not uncommon, because the academic health center is perceived as a powerful hierarchy, with orders and assignments following a chain of authority that goes from the top to the bottom. Nonetheless, there have been some innovative curricular changes at major medical schools in recent times, for example, the integration of problem-based learning throughout all four years at New Mexico, the double-helix curriculum at Rochester based on the biopsychosocial model, and the population health and social medicine inner-city programs at the Sophie Davis State University of New York Medical School, to mention a few.

I build my curricular design on the model created by Wear and Castellani (2000). Professionalism, they argue, "is fostered by students' engagement with significant, integrated experiences with certain kinds of content" (602). They make it clear that professionalism cannot flourish without a sound anchoring of knowledge, skills, and methods. They emphasize "the need for an intellectual widening of the medical curriculum" if professional development is to be enhanced and sustained, and they address, in a straightforward and clear manner, the essential tension between the biomedical paradigm and the "humanistic dimensions of medical practice" (603). If professionalism and its six elements—altruism, accountability, excellence, duty, honor and integrity, and respect for others—are the moral underpinning of medicine, then those must be systematically and thoroughly intertwined throughout the medical school curriculum. In a strict pedagogical sense, Wear and Castellani are talking about content.

They take heed of the dichotomy of medicine as *science* and medicine as *service* that I have tried to confront throughout this thesis. "To ask students to develop compassion, communication skills, and social responsibility within the confines of a biomedical discourse is unrealistic, if not unfair, given the evaluative criteria of success and competency in contemporary medical education." They assert that for learning to be humane, culturally astute, and socially committed, a structure is needed in the form of a curricular innovation that is initiated by the medical school administration, acknowledged by the faculty, and embraced by the students. Such a proposition is a task that is far from easy. Those in charge of teaching medical students have been thoroughly socialized in a biomedical environment in which anything that doesn't fit—sociocultural, economic, and political—is outside scientific scrutiny and based on value judgments.

Their observations highlight the resistance to change by medical school faculty that has been emboldened by a firm belief that medicine, grounded in the basic sciences and learned through practicing in major hospitals that care for the seriously sick, has resulted in the power and prestige of the profession. Wear and Castellani are not inhibited by this challenge and respond by presenting what they call "a Utopian proposal" for a full-spectrum curriculum. They are concerned with continuity from matriculation to licensure, but their main focus is on the four-year medical education curriculum. They frame their approach on Peter Berger's (1965) "sociologic consciousness," which requires rigorous intellectual skills, compassion toward individuals and communities of "disenchanted attitudes," development of a "mobile mind," and a "cosmopolitan attitude" as it applies to medical education. To be a learner you must understand the nature of learning.

Wear and Castellani (2000) maintain that since medical education accepts a reductionistic interpretation of biology as the ultimate foundation of human nature, there is no need to question any of its assumptions. One way of breaking out of that intellectual straitjacket is by being exposed to people and communities outside "safe, harmonious professional relations." I am pleased that the authors see both Bridging the Gap in Philadelphia and RCSIP as examples of becoming immersed in underserved communities. The means for disseminating these wonderful concepts are interspersed throughout the essay in terms of topics (bioethics, literature, philosophy, history of medicine) from the disciplines of the humanities and social sciences, using the modalities of lectures, seminars, and electives. Special emphasis is placed on economic and political considerations (the "marketing" of health care) to be scrutinized in a required senior seminar. Community service experiences would be "woven throughout the four years."

Although extremely useful to the formulation of my proposal, their discussion remains primarily at the theoretical and descriptive level. Let us now return to my first question, How can learning through service remain voluntary and still be required? The answer is, By *tracking*. There is a precedent in the original problem-based learning programs, which demonstrated the efficacy of carefully planned and well organized tracking. At Rush, for example, the problem-based learning track in the preclinical phase was called the *alternative curriculum*. The PBL students—18 of 120—learned independent of the students in the *traditional curriculum*. Other recent educational innovations in medical schools include the *clinical preceptorship* starting in the first year and the *objective clinical examination station* (OCES) as a hands-on way of evaluating clinical skills in the doctor-patient relationship. My proposal is far more radical than those.

The Social Medicine, Community Health, and Human Rights Curriculum

Good tracking requires structure, but too much structure can thwart spontaneity and creativity, two elements that are the essence of the voluntary nature of the kind of community service I am proposing. Participation in the social medicine, community health, and human rights (SMCHHR) track I am proposing is *required* for graduation. But types and levels of participation in the community service and international health components are *voluntary*. Degrees of involvement vary from only one program, to a leadership role (serving on committees), to designing and executing a new program. The alternative option to community service is *epidemiological research,* which can also take various forms, from assisting in an established research project to designing and initiating one of the student's own choice. There are many possibilities here, from learning firsthand what constitutes a randomized clinical trial to conducting a survey of a community or site that is one of the RCSIP-type programs.

The reason I go to such great lengths to preserve the voluntary aspect—giving freely of oneself—is that it promotes humanism. You simply can't require someone to be humanistic, since by its very nature that attribute entrails selflessness, that is, being other-directed. There is a potential humanistic element in the research options as well. The student as epidemiologist will be able to investigate relevant social factors in clinical trails and longitudinal population studies that can be found in almost any clinical research department. For those students who want to survey or observe in neighborhoods where community service activities are ongoing, there is an opportunity to collect data that sheds light on the conditions surrounding the residents' health needs. Besides collecting data for program evaluation, such activities provide the knowledge base for instituting policy. This is not research for its own sake but "action research" to improve existing programs and foster new ones.

There are two significant factors that must be considered in designing the didactic component of SMCHHR, namely, the *stakeholders* and the *sequencing*. The stakeholders are the students, the faculty, and the administration. By sequencing, I mean the continuity and logistic arrangements of the proposed curricular track. I will start with the latter first. A series of focal lectures would run through the first two years, at the start, or pilot phase, six per quarter. A similar series in the form of sociocultural grand rounds would be introduced during the clinical phase, at least two for each core clerkship. These presentations must be exciting as well as informative. Guest speakers of some prominence would add to the attraction. The lecture series needs to correspond to the primary aim of the SMCHHR curriculum, that is, broadening the students' understanding of sociocultural, economic, and political factors and their relation to the health and well-being of collectives of people as manifested in the family, the community, society, and the world.

Readings from the humanities and social sciences would be assigned. History and philosophy will be given special attention. To counter reductionistic thinking, the rudiments of a philosophy of science would be taught in conjunction with the ideas from the Enlightenment that changed Western civilization's notions about the essence of human nature. Themes about health, illness, pain and suffering, and the role of the doctor from classic and modern literature would add a powerful human element and serve to balance the biomedical model that is so rigorously reinforced in traditional medical education. In sum, social factors should be more than population data—the tendency in epidemiology. To complete the course, an essay will be required at the end of the quarter. One approach to the essay would be getting the students to reflect on how the lectures and seminars related to their basic science and pathophysiology studies along with what influence these nonmedical topics had on their perception of themselves as practicing physicians. A final essay in narrative form will be required for graduation.

A key feature would be small-group seminars in which the participants discuss and reflect on their community and research experiences under the guidance of committed faculty advisors. Two two-hour seminars per quarter would be tried at the start. The first hour could serve as a study group during which assigned readings would be discussed and scrutinized. The second hour would focus on service experience and its meaning for the participants. Ideally, two faculty members—one a clinician—would add a broader dimension to the interaction. They would serve as interlocutors to motivate the process. Free and open exchange should be the driving force of these seminars. A class of 120 would have ten such groups. Since the faculty advisors would follow their student cohort for two years, a cadre of at least fifty faculty members should be available for participation. New advisors would be recruited annually. When I initiated the Rush Academic Advisor Program in the 1980s, I had very little trouble recruiting eager faculty members, many of them not too far from finishing their own medical training, who wanted to serve as advisors/mentors to a group of students. (Some senior full professors also applied.) There were so many applicants each year that I had the students help me screen them. The personal satisfaction gained from these experiences can serve as a recruiting mechanism in its own right.

When it comes to the concept of stakeholders, how will students respond to such a proposal? From the community service side, recent surveys of applicants to Rush revealed that RCSIP was mentioned by almost three-fourths of all applicants as a reason for choosing Rush as a potential school for medical training. Of the matriculated applicants almost half indicated that RCSIP was a primary reason for wanting to be a Rush student. RCSIP's reputation was certainly widespread not only among applicants from the metropolitan region but throughout the Midwest and beyond. There is always a pipeline for something especially appealing to idealistic young people. Would a didactic component destroy the essence of volunteering? I don't think so. If designed and planned carefully and perceptively, it would add a missing dimension by placing these experiences in an intellectual context for further study and reflection.

What about the faculty? What must be dealt with is the dilemma I raised earlier; that is, how can such a proposal invade their territory (the existing curriculum) and, at the same time, get them to buy in on a major curricular change? Fortunately, there is already a trend whereby teaching hours in the curriculum of most medical schools are being cut back. In some medical schools there are no longer lectures given in the afternoons. What must be avoided, however, is a return to overstuffing. The resisters, especially the basic science faculty, have to be consulted and made partners in this innovation. Department chairs, who hold positions of power and authority, have to be persuaded that these changes are good for everyone in the long run. The best approach is to involve them and their faculties from the start, not only to endorse the proposal but also to actively engage in it. There are many topics in which they can contribute their knowledge and skills, for example, potential conflicts of interests among scientists at the National Institutes of Health, the role of the basic scientist in evidence-based medicine, and how biology affects behavior and vice versa, to mention a few. A short essay question could be included on examinations asking students to show how social medicine relates to the discipline under study. To illustrate, this would provide the student with an opportunity to show how one could apply a basic science concept (blood sugar) in understanding the symptoms and behavior of an obese person with diabetes living in a community where obesity is the norm or getting people to stop smoking in a disadvantaged community where smoking is one of the few pleasures available.

Without top administration approval, none of this is possible. The task of administrators is enormous. They must cajole the department heads into accepting SMCHHR as an exciting innovation. In particular, this will be especially hard to sell to the basic scientists, and has especially been so since the mapping of the human genome project. The point that must be conveyed is that this is *not* an either/or proposition. An understanding of social and cultural conditions based on meticulous field studies by anthropologists and carefully constructed surveys by sociologists does not detract from the genetic predispositions of people from different "ethnic" origins that correlate with specific illnesses and efforts to treat them. In short, the social construct provides insights regarding issues of compliance, follow-up, and barriers to access to health care.

Without the faculty's support the program is on rocky ground even before it starts. The dean and his or her team of medical educators have to persuade the chairs that medicine's position in society, its sovereignty, its autonomy, and its professionalism are at stake. They need to be shown that this venture offers a unique method for reconnecting medicine to society in a humane as well as a clinical manner. The faculty leaders must become aware that this new curricular track will help bring about that reconnection, and not at the risk of sacrificing the strong biomedical underpinnings that have made American medicine one of the best systems in the world. Additional arguments include the fact that fewer hours teaching means more hours researching, and the new curriculum will focus on promoting the relationship between the "two cultures" not as adversarial but as harmonious.

Of particular importance is the transition to the new track so it complements the traditional one. This will require good planning and clearly defined assignments. A well-thought-out faculty development phase (of probably a year) will need to precede the start of the new track. A team of committed faculty members, under the auspices of the dean's office, would have the duty and responsibility to design, conduct, and implement this learning and development effort. Codirectors (one of them a clinician) will be given the responsibility of overseeing the entire process.

For SMCHHR to work fully as a pedagogical innovation aimed at reaching its goal of fostering humanism in medicine, two other important considerations must be included.

Special effort needs to be invested in recruiting members of minority groups and individuals with working-class backgrounds into medical schools. I am familiar with prematriculation programs geared exclusively toward underrepresented minority students, since I directed one at Rush for a period of seven years.

Since this curriculum is so different, it is necessary to evaluate it as systematically as possible without interfering with the process. A pretest will be administered at matriculation

and a posttest at graduation. The main focus of this survey has three parts: values, perceptions, and expectations. Although attitude scales will be used, open-ended questions will
provide the main source of data. As I have demonstrated, community service participation
can be correlated with academic performance. It will be possible to develop a matrix that
includes the pre- and posttests along with the central components of SMCHHR. A longitudinal schema will be created so the graduates can be followed throughout their careers. A
program evaluator, with personal and technical resources, will be an essential part of the
codirectors' team.

In sum, I am proposing a societal, communal, and humanitarian track that will add a
new and needed dimension to the education of future physicians. I believe that the proposed
innovation, as demonstrated in RCSIP, will breed humanism and social responsibility,
which will serve an important role in getting medicine reconnected to society by addressing issues of social justice and human rights. The real test, of course, is to demonstrate
that students who are products of curricular innovations such as SMCHHR are clinically
competent, ethically concerned, and socially conscious: in sum, what kind of doctors
they become and how they practice medicine to enhance the health of the people. In what
follows, I set out a simple schema of this approach.

The Social Medicine, Community Health, and Human Rights Curriculum

Preclinical Phase

1. Didactics
    Six one-hour lectures quarterly
    Two two-hour small-group discussion sessions quarterly
2. Experiential
    Voluntary community service activities
        Single program
        Committee membership
        Design and implementation of new program
    Other activities
        Epidemiological research
        Clinical research
        Study community service activities

Clinical Phase

Two sociocultural grand rounds per clerkship
Electives

Evaluation

Pre- and posttests (M1–M4)
Final essay (narrative) required for graduation
Enrollment in longitudinal pipeline

Notes

Introduction

1. The original quote, "These are the times that try men's souls," is from *Paine's American Crisis*, no. 1, December 23, 1776.

2. I discuss and dissect the many forms of medical professionalism throughout this book. The following works are some recent examples showing the range of approaches in the struggle for meaning: Swick 2000; Arnold 1997; Rothman 2002; Misch 2002; Wear 2003; American Medical Association Council on Ethical and Judicial Affairs 1996; Wear and Castellani 2000; Inui 2003.

3. In 1910 the Carnegie Foundation hired Abraham Flexner, a professional educator, to conduct a study of medical education in the United States. The Flexner Report (1910) called on American medical schools to enact higher admission and graduate standards and to adhere strictly to the protocols of mainstream science in their teaching and research. The first two years of medical education were to be anchored in basic sciences and the pathology of disease. On the basis of this foundation, doctors-in-training would now be able to apply their knowledge and skills to patients in the clinics and hospitals and after a total of four years' training would be certified as medical doctors. As a result of these standards nearly half the existing medical schools were closed. An excellent summary of the Flexner Report can be found on Wikipedia (http://wikipedia.org/wiki/Flexner.Report).

4. The Health of the Public: An Academic Challenge, sponsored by the Pew Charitable Trust, the Robert Wood Johnson Foundation, and the Rockefeller Foundation, consisted of thirty-three participating academic health centers in the United States and Canada (Rush was one). These initiatives were dedicated to advancing the "population perspective" through community partnerships, curricular reform, and collaboration among health professions. The Health of the Public developed criteria for program design and execution that including ways of achieving change *within* the academic health center as well as ways of achieving change in the academic health center's role *in the community*. The program ended in 2001 after more than a decade of activity.

5. Paul Farmer was the driving force behind the creation of Partners in Health (PIH). PIH is a Boston-based nonprofit health care program dedicated to providing "a preferential option for the poor" that was founded in 1987, two years after the Clinique Bon Sauveur was set up in Cange, Haiti, to deliver health care to the residents of the mountainous Central Plateau. PIH, now directed by Ophelia Dahl along with the involvement of Thomas White and Todd McCormack, has since expanded its operations to eight other sites in Haiti and five additional countries and has launched a number of other initiatives. The PIH model of care is based on partnering with poor communities to combat disease and poverty. It strives to bring the best of Western medicine to the poorest of the poor by establishing long-term partnerships with local sister organizations. Zanmi Lasante in Haiti is PIH's flagship project—the oldest, largest, most ambitious, and the most replicated. Besides Haiti, PIH serves Peru, Russia, and Rwanda, especially in the treatment of tuberculosis and HIV/AIDS. In addition, PIH has supported projects in Chiapas, Mexico, and Guatemala.

To date, Farmer has been the recipient of two MacArthur Foundation "genius" awards. One of his original partners, Jim Kim, a physician, has also received one of the MacArthur awards. All the funding goes into supporting the program.

6. The epicenter of sociology in America is found in the so-called Chicago school. Founded by Albion Small in 1892, the Department of Sociology at the University of Chicago attracted brilliant thinkers of the post-Enlightenment period such as Robert Park and Ernest Burgess who were interested primarily in humans as social beings and in their normative behavior. Instead of following in the tradition of theoretical and historic treatises conceptualized by Emile Durkheim and Max Weber, they had a focus on field studies and empirical research, for which the Chicago school became celebrated. The city of Chicago became their laboratory. Park was concerned with industrial organizations and what he called the moral order of social aggregates, which included families, communities, and large urban areas. Burgess created the "concentric ring diagram" of Chicago, which ushered in the field of urban sociology. In the second phase of the Chicago school, the perspective on social behavior and human ecology was expanded and new areas of research, among them deviant behavior and social movements, were delineated. For well-researched documentation of the Chicago school, see Bulmer 1984.

7. *New University Thought* was a radical journal started by graduate students at the University of Chicago in 1960. Its "mission statement" reads: "We, young intellectuals, students, and professionals, founded *New University Thought* (1961) because we were dissatisfied with what we saw. The gigantic resources of the academic world seemed to be focused on everything but the critical questions in our society" (inside front cover).

8. Rush Medical College is named after Benjamin Rush, a signer of the Declaration of Independence and George Washington's physician. The college, first chartered in 1837, was one of the few medical schools in the Midwest that met the high standards Abraham Flexner set in 1910 for his monumental study of American medical education. At the very end of the nineteenth century, Rush became part of the new and highly regarded University of Chicago, which offered Rush research facilities and a university setting. The relationship lasted forty-four years. When this affiliation ended, the Rush charter was deactivated, but in 1969, with the dearth of physicians and the desperate need for more medical schools, Rush Medical College reactivated its charter and its new home was Presbyterian–St. Luke's Hospital on Chicago's West Side. (*Rush* was added to the name of the medical center when the medical school was activated.) The medical center continued to expand and established a college of nursing (which awards PhD degrees), a college in the health sciences, a graduate college, a health systems management school, and training in the allied health fields. Student enrollment remains close to fifteen hundred. In 2004 the institution changed its name to Rush University Medical Center.

9. In a speech at the University of Michigan on May 22, 1964, President Lyndon B. Johnson proclaimed, "I intend to establish working groups to prepare a series of conferences and meetings—on the cities, on natural beauty, on the quality of education, and on other emerging challenges. From these studies, we will begin to set the course toward the Great Society." The most ambitious and controversial part of the Great Society was the War on Poverty. The centerpiece was the 1964 Economic Opportunities Act, which created the Office of Economic Opportunity to oversee a variety of community-based antipoverty programs. To address the health care needs of poor and disadvantaged communities, a series of free neighborhood

health centers were created. The Mile Square Health Center was one of the first of these established in the country.

10. The Holmes County Health Research Project (HCHRP) was designed to carry out an extensive investigation of the relationship between the physical and social environment of a poverty-stricken, rural, black population and its endemic disease patterns in 1969. The black people of Holmes County were among the first predominantly rural populations to become active in the civil rights movement in the early 1960s. In 1967 they formed the Milton Olive III Memorial Corporation (MOMC). The HCHRP was unprecedented for a health research proposal because MOMC was the grantee; an indigenous schoolteacher was the principal investigator; a network of professional, unpaid consultants accepted responsibility for the research design, execution, and evaluation; a staff of local people were trained to perform program tasks; and the aim of the research was instituting a series of intervention efforts that would eventually lead to full-scale community development programs.

Chapter 2   Clinics Serving the Poor and Homeless

1. This description is from "A Short History of Englewood," by Maureen Spokes (http://people.virginia.edu/%7Emrs8t/englewood).
2. These statistics are taken from the Chicago Community Area Health and Demographic Data, collected and organized by the University of Chicago in conjunction with the Chicago Health Department.
3. Vital statistics come from the Chicago Community Area Health and Demographic Data base.
4. Historical information on Pilsen and Little Village comes from many sources, chiefly "A Primer: Little Village and Pilsen," by Alexander Russo, available at www.catalyst-chicago.org, and two of seventy-seven official community areas, the Near West Side, Chicago, and South Lawndale, Chicago, from Wikipedia, the free encyclopedia on the Internet.
5. The Illinois Medical District, with Chicago Technical Park, has its own Web site (www.imdc.org), which offers detailed information about the operation, including facts on more than fifty thousand direct and indirect jobs. Information on the Franciscan House of Mary and Joseph can be obtained through their e-mail address: mail@franoutreach.org.
6. CommunityHealth also has its own Web site (www.communityhealth.org), which is updated on a regular basis. Sociodemographic data for the Near West Side can be found through the database developed by the Chicago Health Department. These data can be accessed at http://chas.uchicago.edu/data/atlas/ca68.html.

Chapter 3   The New Faces of AIDS

1. Ounce of Prevention is a nonprofit organization in Chicago that invests in the healthy development of infants and children through such endeavors as family-focus programs, research, policy analysis, and advocacy.

Chapter 4   Community-Based Grassroots Programs

Bridging the Gap is a voluntary student community service program administered jointly by seven academic health centers in the Commonwealth of Pennsylvania. It combines health-related service in underserved communities with training community-responsive health and social service students working in coordination with health professional mentors.

1. HUD can be traced back to the New Deal as part of the U.S. Housing Act of 1937. HUD's mandate is to increase homeownership, support community development, and increase affordable housing that is free from discrimination.
2. Governor Henry Horner is credited with establishing several programs to aid the economically disadvantaged.
3. Monsignor Gerardi was the driving force behind the project Recovery of Historical Memory (REMHI), created to shed light on the war's human rights violations. Activists said the murder was a direct reply to the presentation of the REMHI, which blamed the army for at least 90 percent of the massacres and other killings and human rights violations during the war.

Chapter 5   The Community Today, Tomorrow the World

1. Médecins sans frontières (MSF) is an international independent medical humanitarian organization that delivers emergency aid to people affected by armed conflicts, epidemics, natural and human-made disasters, and exclusion from health care in more than seventy countries. It was founded by a group of French doctors in 1971 and today has an international network with sections in nineteen countries. The U.S. section was founded in 1990. MSF was awarded the 1999 Noble Peace Prize.
2. The quotes that follow are taken from "The Roots of Reform," an excellent overview of Professor Nussbaum's conceptualization for "cultivating humanity" that appeared in the *University of Chicago Magazine* (Nussbaum 1997b).

Chapter 6   Looking for Meaning

1. The Medical Schools Objectives Project report has become a watershed for reform in contemporary medical education. The four major attributes of a clinically competent and compassionate physician are stated in terms of the imperative *must*, and the report advances the notion that besides being knowledgeable and skillful, today's physician must be *altruistic* and *dutiful.*

Chapter 9   Nurturing Idealism, Advancing Humanism,
**   and Planning Reform**

1. For more on Paul Farmer, see the introduction, note 5.
2. In *evidence-based medicine*, the standards of evidence gained from the scientific method to certain aspects of medical practice that depend on *rational* assessments of the risks and benefits of treatments are applied more uniformly. *Information systems*, as applied to the practice of medicine, is the name of a method for computerizing a patient's physical evaluation and laboratory test results to avoid omissions and redundancies. The clinical judgments about the patient's condition and the data for assessment are strictly biomedical. The catch phrase of *translational research* is "from the bench to the bedside." What is left out is the fact that the patient in the bed is a person who is a member of a family or social group that is part of a community with values, attitudes, and beliefs.
3. SCHIP is jointly financed by the federal and state governments and is administered by the states. Within broad federal guidelines, each state determines the design of its program, eligibility groups, benefit packages, payment levels of coverage, and administrative and operating procedures. Program benefits became available on October 1, 1997.
4. Lake Research Partners is a national public opinion and political strategy research firm. The organization is a principal strategy group for the Democratic Party and

provides tacticians to a wide range of advocacy organizations, nonprofit organizations, and foundations.

Chapter 10   A Personal Reflection: The Staying Power of the Call of Service

1. I use the term advisedly primarily because it tends to imply a homogeneous group, usually white and middle class, that is, a "product" of a public culture. A good example of this narrow interpretation as applied to academic medicine can be found in J. Bickel and A. J. Brown 2005. For a serious analysis, see Ortner 2006.

Bibliography

Accreditation Council for Graduate Medical Education. 1999. "Enhancing Residency Education through Outcomes Assessment." ACGME Outcomes Project. Chicago. http://www.acgme.org/outcome/implement/rsvp.asp.

Agee, James, and Walker Evans. 1960. *Let Us Now Praise Famous Men.* Introduction by John Hershey. Boston: Houghton Mifflin.

Allport, G. 1962. "Psychological Models for Guidance." *Harvard Educational Review* 32, no. 4:373–381.

American Board of Internal Medicine. 2001. "Project Professionalism." Philadelphia.

American College of Physicians. 2006. "The Impending Collapse of Primary Care Medicine and Its Implication for the State of the Nation's Health Care." Report from the American College of Physicians. Philadelphia.

American Medical Association, Council on Ethical and Judicial Affairs. 1996. "Code of Medical Ethics: Current Opinions with Annotations." Chicago.

Angel, M. 2004. *The Truth about the Drug Companies: How They Deceive Us and What to Do about It.* New York: Random House.

Arnold, L. 1997. "Assessing Professional Behavior: Yesterday, Today, and Tomorrow." *Academic Medicine* 72:941–952.

Bardack, M., and S. Thompson. 1992. "Model Prenatal Program of Rush Medical College at St. Basil's Free People's Clinic, Chicago." *Public Health Reports* 108:161–165.

Becker, H., B. Greer, E. C. Hughes, and A. Strauss. 1961. *Boys in White: Student Culture in Medical School.* Chicago: University of Chicago Press.

———. 2002. *Boys in White: Student Culture in Medical School,* rev. ed. New Brunswick, NJ: Transaction.

Bellah, R., R. Madsen, W. Sullivan, A. Swidler, and S. Tipton. 1986. *Habits of the Heart: Individualism and Commitment in American Life.* New York: Harper and Row.

Berger, P. 1965. *Invitation to Sociology.* New York: Anchor Books.

Besteman, C., and H. Gusterson, eds. 2005. *Why America's Top Pundits Are Wrong: Anthropologists Talk Back.* Berkeley and Los Angeles: University of California Press.

Bickel, J., and A. J. Brown. 2005. "Generation X: Implications for Faculty Recruitment and Development in Academic Health Centers." *Academic Medicine* 80:205–210.

Bloom, B. S. 1956. *Taxonomy of Educational Objectives: Cognitive Domain.* New York: David McKay.

Bloom, S. W. 1988. "Structure and Ideology in Medical Education: An Analysis of Resistance to Change." *Journal of Health and Social Behavior* 29, no. 4:294–306.

Brooks, D. 2007. "The Next Culture War." Op-ed, *New York Times,* June 12.

Bulmer, M. 1984. *The Chicago School of Sociology: Institutionalization, Diversity, and the Rise of Social Research.* Chicago: University of Chicago Press.

Carey, B. 2007. "This is Your Life (and How You Tell It)." Op-ed, *New York Times,* May 22.

Charon, R. 1993. "The Narrative Road to Empathy." In H. M. Spiro, ed., *Empathy and the Practice of Medicine: Beyond Pills and the Scalpel.* New Haven: Yale University Press.

Chicago Community Area Health and Demographic Data, University of Chicago in conjunction with the Chicago Health Department. Center for Health Administration Studies, University of Chicago. http://www.chas.uchicago.edu/healthdata/atlas.

Christakis, N. A. 1992. *Interim Report of the Acadia Institute on Undergraduate Medical Education.* Philadelphia: Medical College of Pennsylvania.

———. 1995a. *Implicit Purposes of Proposal to Reform American Medical Education.* Philadelphia: Medical College of Pennsylvania Press.

———. 1995b. "The Similarity and Frequency of Proposals to Reform U.S. Medical Education." *JAMA* 274, no. 9:706–711.

Clendinen, D. 2003. "AIDS after 'Angels': Not Gone, Not Forgotten." Op-ed, *New York Times,* December 16.

Cohen, P. 2004. "Forget Lonely. Life Is Healthier at the Top." *New York Times,* May 15.

Cohen, S. 2005. "A Day in the Life of the Homeless." *New York Times Magazine,* February 27.

Cohn, J. 2007. *Sick: The Untold Story of America's Health Care Crisis—and the People Who Pay the Price.* New York: HarperCollins.

Coles, R. 1990. *The Call of Stories: Teaching and the Moral Imagination.* Boston: Mariner Books.

———. 1993. *The Call of Service: A Witness to Idealism.* New York: Houghton Mifflin.

———. 2003. "The Moral Education of Medical Students." In R. Coles, R. Testa, and J. O'Donnell, eds., *A Life in Medicine: A Literary Anthropology.* New York: New Press. Originally published in *Academic Medicine* 73, no. 1:55–57.

Community-Campus Partnerships for Health. 1996. Mission statement. http://www/cpph.info.

Connolly, C. 2005. "Data Show Scourge of Hospital Infections." *Washington Post,* July 13.

Critical Challenges: Revitalizing the Health Professions for the Twenty-first Century. 1995. Third report of the Pew Professions Commission. San Francisco: Center for the Health Professions.

Cruess, R. L., S. R. Cruess, and S. E. Johnston. 1999. "Renewing Professionalism: An Opportunity for Medicine." *Academic Medicine* 74:878–884.

Cruess, S. R., and R. L. Cruess. 1997. "Teaching Professionalism." *British Journal of Medicine* 314:1674–1677.

Declaration on Public Health, Peace and Human Rights. 2001. Skopje, Macedonia. Stability Pact of Southeastern Europe. December.

Doctors without Borders (Médecins Sans Frontières). http://www.doctorswithoutborders.org.

Du Bois, W. E. B. 1903. *The Souls of Black Folk.* Boulder, CO: Paradigm, 2004.

Durant, Will, and Ariel Durant. 1993. *The Lessons of History.* New York: MJF Books.

Eckenfels, E. 1976. "Community Control, Action Research, and Program Efficacy: An Overview of the Holmes County, Mississippi Health Research Project." Report submitted to the National Center for Health Service Research and Development, Department of Health, Education, and Welfare, Washington, DC.

———. 1988. *Basic Principles and Guidelines of the Rush Academic Advisor Program.* Chicago: Rush University Medical Center.

———. 1993. "Student-Faculty Collaboration to Enhance Community Health." In W. Skelton and M. Osterweis, eds., *Promoting Community Health: The Role of Academic Health Centers.* Washington, DC: Association of Academic Health Centers.

———. 1994. "The Rush–Henry Horner Homes Pediatric Asthma Pilot Program: Phase I." Prepared for Rush Community Service Intitiatives Program, Rush University Medical Center, Chicago.

———. 1995. "A Sociodemographic Profile of Guatemalans in Chicago." Paper presented at the Second Symposium on Latin American Human Rights, University of Chicago, October.

Eckenfels, E. 1996. "Health Manpower Development: An American Experience." WHO Conference, Delphi, Greece.

———. 1997. "Contemporary Medical Students' Quest for Self-Fulfillment through Community Service." *Academic Medicine* 72:1043–1050.

———. 2000a. "The Case for Keeping Community Service Voluntary: Narratives from the Rush Community Service Initiatives Program." In D. Wear and J. Bickel, eds., *Education for Professionalism: Creating a Culture of Humanism in Medical Education.* Iowa City: University of Iowa Press.

———. 2000b. Towards a Humanitarian Cause. Session at the Ninth International Health in Medical Education Conference, Vancouver, BC, March.

———. 2001. "Learning about Ethics: The Cardinal Rule of the Clinical Experience." *Journal of Medical Education* 35:716–717.

———. 2002. "Vulnerability Reduction in the United States: A Personal Perspective." *Croatian Medical Journal* 43, no. 2:157–162.

———. 2004. "The Struggle for the Soul of Medicine." *Annals of Behavioral Science in Medical Education* 10:34–38.

Eckenfels, E., and W. Addington. 1999. "Student-Generated Initiatives for Community Service and International Health: Broadening the Vision of the Academic Health Center after the Second Millennium." Universities and the Health of the Disadvantaged: A Global Conference, Tucson, Arizona, July.

Eckenfels, E., C. Baier, K. Turner-Roan, and A. Sanchez. 1994. "Enhancing the Learning and Development of Medical Students through Community Service." In *Effective Learning, Effective Teaching, Effective Service: The Voice from the Field on Improving Education through Community-Service Learning.* Washington, DC: Youth Serving Policy.

Eckenfels, E., R. Blacklow, and G. Gotterer. 1984. "Medical Student Counseling: The Rush Medical College Advisor Program." *Academic Medicine* 59:573–581.

Eckenfels, E., and L. Landry. 1962. "A 1961 Peace Walk." *New University Thought* 2, no. 3:92–97.

Ehrenreich, B. 2001. *Nickel and Dimed.* New York: Henry Holt.

Epstein, H. 2003. "Enough to Make You Sick?" *New York Times Magazine,* 12 October.

Evans, J. 1992. "The Health of the Public Approach to Medical Education." *Academic Medicine* 67:719–723.

Fadiman, A. 1997. *The Spirit Catches You and You Fall Down.* New York: Farrar, Straus and Giroux.

Fanon, F. 1963. *The Wretched of the Earth.* New York: Grove Press.

Farmer, P. 2003. *Pathologies of Power: Health, Human Rights, and the War on Poverty.* Berkeley and Los Angeles: University of California Press.

Farmer, P., and A. Kleinman. 1989. "AIDS as Human Suffering." *Daedalus* 118, no. 2:135–160.

Flexner, A. 1910. *Medical Education in the United States and Canada.* New York: Carnegie Foundation for the Advancement of Teaching.

Fox, R. 1979. *Essays in Medical Sociology: Health, Medicine, and Society.* New York: John Wiley and Sons.

Fox, R. 1990. "Training in Care Competence: The Perennial Problem in North American Medical Education." In H. Hendrie and C. Lloyd, eds., *Educating Competent and Humane Physicians.* Bloomington: Indiana University Press.

Fox, R., and J. Swazey. 1984. "Medical Morality Not Bioethics in China and the United States." *Perspectives in Biology and Medicine* 27:336–340.

Franciscan House of Mary and Joseph. (An emergency overnight shelter with 250 beds.) http://www.franoutreach.org.

Freidson, E. 1970. *Profession of Medicine: A Study in the Sociology of Applied Knowledge.* New York: Dodd, Mead.

Gardner, H., M. Csikszentmihalyi, and W. Damon. 2001. *Good Work: When Excellence and Ethics Meet.* New York: Basic Books.

Gawande, A. 2002. *Complications: A Surgeon's Notes on an Imperfect Science.* New York: Picador.

General Assembly of the United Nations. 1948. The Universal Declaration of Human Rights, adopted, December 10, Article 25. http://www.un.org/Overview/rights.html.

Gerth, H., and C. W. Mills. 1958. *From Max Webber: Essays in Sociology.* New York: Oxford University Press.

Giroux, H. 2000. "Insurgent Multiculturalism and the Promise of Pedagogy." In E. Duarte and S. Smith, eds., *Foundational Perspectives in Multicultural Education.* New York: Longman.

Good, B. 1994. *Medicine, Rationality, and Experience: An Anthropological Perspective.* New York: Cambridge University.

Goulet, D. 1971. "An Ethical Model for the Study of Values." *Education, Participation, and Power: Essays in Theory and Practice.* Special issue of *Harvard Educational Review.* Reprint series no. 10:35–57.

Groopman, J. 2007. *How Doctors Think.* Boston: Houghton Mifflin.

Hafferty, F. 1998. "Beyond Curriculum Reform: Confronting Medicine's Hidden Curriculum." *Academic Medicine* 73:403–407.

———. 2000. "In Search of a Lost Cord: Professionalism and Medical Education's Hidden Curriculum". In D. Wear and J. Bickel, eds., *Education for Professionalism: Creating a Culture of Humanism in Medical Education.* Iowa City: University of Iowa Press.

Hafferty, F., and R. Franks. R. 1994. "The Hidden Curriculum, Ethics Teaching, and the Structure of Medical Education". *Academic Medicine* 69:861–871.

Halpern, Jodi. 1993. "Empathy: Using Resonance Emotions in the Service of Curiosity." In H. M. Spiro, ed., *Empathy and the Practice of Medicine: Beyond Pills and the Scalpel.* New Haven: Yale University Press.

Hancock, T. 1993. "Healthy Communities: The Role of the Academic Health Center." In W. Skelton and M. Osterweis, eds., *Promoting Community Health: The Role of the Academic Health Center.* Washington, DC: Association of Academic Health Centers.

Harris, G. "Doctors Back Ban on Drug Companies' Gifts" *New York Times,* January 26, 2006.

Havel, V. 1994. "The Measure of the New Man." Op-ed, *New York Times,* July 8.

"Health of the Public: The Evolution of a Movement." 1996. *Challenge: Academe and the Health of the Public* 6, no. 1.

Health Professional Schools in Service to the Nation (HPSISN). 1996. San Francisco: Center for Health Professions, September 23.

Horton, R. 2003. *Health Wars: On the Global Front Lines of Modern Medicine.* New York: New York Review of Books.

———. 2007. "What's Wrong with Doctors." *New York Review of Books* 54, no. 9:16–20.

Howell, J. D. 1992. "Lowell T. Coggeshall and American Medical Education, 1901–1987." *Academic Medicine* 67, no. 11:711–742.

Illinois Medical District and Chicago Technical Park. http://www.imdc.org.

Institute of Medicine. 2001. *Crossing the Quality Chasm: A New Health Care System for the Twenty-first Century.* Washington, DC: National Academy Press.

———. 2002. *Unequal Treatment: Confronting Racial and Ethnic Disparities in Healthcare.* Washington, DC: National Academies Press.

Inui, T. 2003. *A Flag in the Wind: Education for Professionalism in Medicine.* Washington, DC: American Association of Medical Colleges.

———. 2004. "Viewpoint: Educating for Professionalism in Medicine." *AAMC Reporter,* September.

Kaiser Daily Health Policy Report. 2004. "82M U.S. Residents Uninsured at Some Point over Last Two Years." June 16. http://www.kaisernetwork.org.

———. 2006. "President Bush Signs FY 2006 Budget Reconciliation Measure with Reductions for Medicare, Medicaid." February 9.

Kaufman, Arthur. 2001. An interview. *Education for Health* 14, no. 1:219–224.

Kidder, T. 2003. *Mountains beyond Mountains: The Quest of Dr. Paul Farmer, a Man Who Would Cure the World.* New York: Random House.

Kleinman, A. 1988. *The Illness Narratives: Suffering, Healing, and the Human Condition.* New York: Basic Books.

———. 1995. *Writing on the Margin.* Berkeley and Los Angeles: University of California Press.

Kolb, D. 1984. *Experiential Learning: Experience as the Source of Learning and Development.* Englewood Cliffs, NJ: Prentice-Hall.

Kotlowitz, A. 1992. *There Are No Children Here: The Story of Two Boys Growing Up in the Other America.* New York: Random House.

Krugman, P. 2007a. "Edwards Gets It Right." Op-ed, *New York Times,* February 9.

———. 2007b. "First Do Less Harm." Op-ed, *New York Times,* January 5.

Lake Research Partners. http://www.lakesnellperry.com.

Lakoff, G. 2004. *Don't Think of an Elephant! Know Your Values and Frame the Debate.* White River Junction, VT: Chelsea Green.

Landes, D. 1998. *The Wealth and Poverty of Nations: Why Some Are So Rich and Some Are So Poor.* New York: W. W. Norton.

Larson, E. 2004. *The Devil in the White City.* New York: Vintage Books.

Levitt, S. D., and S. J. Dubner. 2005. *Freaknomics: A Rogue Economist Explores the Hidden Side of Everything.* New York: William Morrow.

Lewis, O. 2002. "The Culture of Poverty." In G. Gmelch and W. Zenner, eds., *Urban Life: Readings in the Anthropology of the City.* Long Grove, IL: Waveland Press.

Ludmerer, Kenneth M. 2004. *Time to Heal: American Medical Education from the Turn of the Century to the Era of Managed Care.* New York: Oxford University Press.

Lustig, S. 1994. "The AIDS Prevention Magic Show: Preventing the Tragic with Magic." *Public Health Reports* 109:204–208.

Margasak, L. 2006. "Edwards Touts Investments in Health Care." *Washington Post,* December 31.

Marmot, M. 2004. *The Status Syndrome: How Social Standing Affects Our Health and Longevity.* New York: Times Books.

Martinez, R. 2000. "Toward an Ethics of Authenticity." In D. Wear and J. Bickel, eds., *Education for Professionalism: Creating a Culture of Humanism in Medical Education.* Iowa City: University of Iowa Press.

Mathieu, A. 2004. "Understanding the Debate on Medical Education Research: A Sociological Perspective." *Academic Medicine* 79, no. 10:948–954.

McCanne, D. 2007. "Opposing Views: State Plans Miss the Point." January 16. http://capa.pnhp.org.

McKersie, R. C. 2005. *In the Foothills of Medicine: A Young Doctor's Journey from the Inner City of Chicago to the Mountains of Nepal.* New York: iUniverse.

"Medical Professionalism in the New Millennium: A Physician Charter." 2002. Project of ABIM Foundation, ACP-ASIM Foundation and European Federation of Internal Medicine. *Annals of Internal Medicine* 136, no. 3:243–246.

Medical School Objectives Project. 1998. "Learning Objectives for Medical Students' Education: Guidelines for Medical Schools." Washington, DC: American Association of Medical Colleges.

Michaels, W. B. 2007. *The Trouble with Diversity: How We Learn to Love Identity and Ignore Inequality.* New York: Metropolitan Books.

Mills, C. W. 1959. *The Sociological Imagination.* New York: Oxford University Press.

Miringoff, M., and M. F. Miringoff. 1999. *The Social Health of the Nation: How America Is Really Doing.* New York: Oxford.

Misch, D. 2002. "Evaluating Physicians' Professionalism and Humanism: The Case for Humanism 'Connoisseurs.'" *Academic Medicine* 77:489–495.

New University Thought. 1961. Editorial, vol. 1, no. 3. Chicago.

Nussbaum, M. 1997a. *Cultivating Humanity: A Classical Defense of Reform in Liberal Education.* Cambridge, MA: Harvard University Press.

———. 1997b. "The Roots of Reform." *University of Chicago Magazine,* December.

———. 2001. *Upheavals of Thought: The Intelligence of Emotions.* New York: Cambridge University Press.

O'Neil, E. 2007. "Centering on . . . Proposed Reforms." http://www.futurehealth. ucsf.edu/fromthedirector.html.

Ortner, S. B. 2006. *Anthropology and Social Theory: Culture, Power, and the Acting Subject.* Durham: Duke University Press.

O'Toole, J. 1995. "The Story of Ethics: Narratives as a Means for Ethical Understanding and Action." Pulse, *JAMA* 273, no. 7:1387–1390.

Paine, T. 1776. *Common Sense.* Philadelphia: W. and T. Bradford.

Palmer, P. 1997. *The Courage to Teach: Exploring the Inner Landscape of a Teacher's Life.* San Francisco: Jossey-Bass.

Parsons, T. 1951. *The Social System.* Glencoe, IL: Free Press.

Partners in Health. http://www.pih.org.

Patterson, O. 2006. "The Last Race Problem." *New York Times,* December 30.

Pear, R. 2004. "Health Spending at Record High." *New York Times,* January 9.

Perspective. 1996. World Health Organization Conference, Delphi, Greece, May.

Poole, I. J. 2007. "Universal Care: Watch Your Language." http://www.tompaine.com. Accessed February 27.

"Project 3000 by 2000—Racial and Ethnic Diversity in US Medical Schools." 1994. Sounding Board. *New England Journal of Medicine* 331:472–476.

Putnam, R. 2000. *Bowling Alone: The Collapse and Revival of American Community.* New York: Simon and Schuster.

Reed, J. 2002. "More Control and Less Negative Energy." In R. Couto, *To Give Their Gifts: Health, Community, and Democracy.* Nashville: Vanderbilt University Press.

Relman, A. S. 2007. *A Second Opinion: Rescuing America's Health Care.* New York: Public Affairs.

Richards, R. 1996. *Building Partnerships: Educating Professionals for the Community They Serve.* San Francisco: Jossey-Bass.

Rorty, R. 1998. *Achieving Our Country.* Cambridge: Harvard University Press.

Rose, G. 1992. *The Strategy of Preventive Medicine.* Oxford: Oxford University Press.

Rothman, D. 2002. "Medical Professionalism: Focusing on the Real Issues." *New England Journal of Medicine* 342:1284–1286.

Rumi, Jelaluddin. 1997. *The Essential Rumi.* Translated by Coleman Barks. Edison, NJ: Castle Books.

Rush, B. 1786. "Thoughts upon the Model of Education Proper in a Republic." Rush University Medical Center Archives, Chicago.

Russo, A. 2003. "A Primer: Little Village and Pilsen." http://www.catalyst-chicago.org.

Schmidt, H. 1993. "Foundation of Problem-Based Learning: Some Explanatory Notes." *Medical Education* 27:422–432.

Schroeder, S. 1992. "The Troubled Profession: Is Medicine's Glass Half Full or Half Empty?" *Annals of Internal Medicine* 116:583–592.

Schroeder, S., J. Zones, and J. Showstack. 1989. "Academic Medicine as Public Trust." *JAMA* 262:803–812.

Seifer, S. 1998. "Service Learning: Community Campus Partnerships for Health Professional Education." *Academic Medicine* 73:273–277.

Sen, A. 2004. "Passage to China." *New York Review of Books* 51:61–65.

Shipler, D. 2004a. "Total Poverty Awareness." Op-ed, *New York Times,* February 21.

———. 2004b. *The Working Poor: Invisible in America.* New York: Alfred Knopf.

Showstack, J, O. Fein, and D. Ford. 1992. "The Health of the Public: The Academic Response." *JAMA* 267:2497–2502.

"Slow Medicine Puts Med Students on Fast Track to High Touch Care." 1992. *American Hospital Association News,* March.

Soros, G. 2002. *On Globalization.* New York: Perseus Books for *Public Affairs.*

Spokes, M. 2004. "A Short History of Englewood." m.spokes@verizon.net.

Starr, P. 1982. *The Social Transformation of American Medicine.* New York: Basic Books.

Suttles, G. D. 1968. *The Social Order of the Slums: Ethnicity and Territory in the Inner City.* Chicago: University of Chicago Press.

Swartz, D. 1997. *Culture and Power: The Sociology of Pierre Bourdieu.* Chicago: University of Chicago Press.

Swazey, J. P., et al., eds. n.d. *Undergraduate Medical Education: In Search of Reform with Change.* Interim report of the Acadia Institute and the Medical College of Pennsylvania Project on Undergraduate Medical Education. Philadelphia: Medical College of Pennsylvania.

Swick, H. 2000. "Toward a Normative Definition of Medical Professionalism." *Academic Medicine* 75:612–616.

Taylor, C. 1992. *The Ethics of Authenticity.* Cambridge: Harvard University Press.

Tess, J., C. Baier, E. Eckenfels, and R. Yogev. 1997. "Medical Students Act as Big Brothers/Sisters to Support HIV-Infected Children's Psychosocial Needs." *Archives of Pediatric and Adolescent Medicine* 151:476–481.

Top 10 Health Policy Stories/Issues. 2004. Commonwealth Fund, December 17. http://www.commonwealthfund.org/aboutus/aboutus_show.htm?doc_id = 252816.

"Townsend Letter for Doctors and Patients: Stress and Illness." 2004. Townsend Letter Group. http://www.townsendletter.com.

Tuton, L., C. Siegel, and T. Campbell. 2000. "Bridging the Gap: Community Health Internship Program." In D. Wear and J. Bickel, eds., *Education for Professionalism: Creating a Culture of Humanism in Medical Education.* Iowa City: University of Iowa Press.

Wear, D. 1997. "Professional Development of Medical Students: Problems and Promises." *Academic Medicine* 72:1056–1062.

———. 2003. "Insurgent Multiculturalism: Rethinking How and Why We Teach Culture in Medical Education." *Academic Medicine* 78:549–554.

Wear, D., and B. Castellani. 2000. "The Development of Professionalism: Curriculum Matters." *Academic Medicine* 75:602–611.

Weiss, K., P. Gergen, and T. Hodgson. 1992. "An Economic Evaluation of Asthma in the United States." *New England Journal of Medicine* 326, no. 13:862–871.

White, K. 1992. "Health Care Organizations: An Epidemiological Perspective." In *Health Services Research: An Anthology.* Washington, DC: Pan American Health Organization.

Whitehead, A. 1978. *Progress and Reality.* Chicago: Free Press.

Wills, G. 2000. *Papal Sins.* New York: Doubleday.

Wilson, W. J. 1987. *The Truly Disadvantaged: The Inner City, the Underclass, and Public Policy.* Chicago: University of Chicago Press.

Woolland, R. 2003. "Citizenship of Medical Schools." *The Network: Towards Unity in Health* 22:18.

World Health Reports. 2000. *Health Systems: Improving Performance.* Geneva: World Health Organization.

Zakaria, F. 2005. "The Assassins' Gate: Occupational Hazard." *New York Times,* October 3.

Index

Note: Page numbers followed by "t" refer to tables and charts

127, 176–180; public relations aspects of, 21, 26, 131, 184; skills developed through, 9, 18, 20, 35–41, 46–47, 50, 52, 98, 113–114, 116, 128*t*, 129–130, 134; unique characteristics of, 9–10, 15, 153. *See also* RSIHM

Rush Medical College (Chicago), 188n8; administration of, 12, 100, 130, 136, 158, 181; alternative curriculum at, 127, 183; Department of Behavioral Science in, 19; Department of Cardiology in, 19; Department of Dermatology in, 19; Department of Family Medicine in, 25–26, 45, 49; Department of Immunology in, 68, 83; Department of Infectious Diseases in, 19; Department of Neurology in, 19; Department of Obstetrics and Gynecology in, 35–36; Department of Ophthalmology in, 19; Department of Pediatrics in, 83; Department of Pharmacology in, 19; Department of Preventive Medicine in, 8, 19, 21, 33, 54, 58, 69; Department of Radiology in, 19; Eckenfels hired by, 7–8; goals of, 129; in Health of the Public program, 29, 187n4; RCSIP as factor in medical students' choice of, 17, 50, 52, 168, 184; RCSIP as recognized part of, 10, 131, 168; RCSIP's clinics located near, 62; RCSIP students' ambiguous relation to, 25–26, 41–42; reputation of, in surrounding neighborhood, 24–26, 49; tests at, 35–36. *See also* faculty; medical education; Rush Community Service Initiatives Program (RCSIP); Rush University Medical Center; students

Rush Pediatric AIDS Support Program, 68–73, 77, 78, 113, 119*t*, 124, 125*t*, 166, 167

Rush Prenatal Program (St. Basil's Free People's Clinic), 27, 34–36, 40–41, 43, 63, 119*t*, 121, 122*t*, 123

Rush–Presbyterian–St. Luke's Medical Center (Chicago), 25, 36, 188n8

Rush Students for International Health and Medicine (RSIHM), 97–107

Rush University Medical Center, 168, 188n8. *See also* Rush Medical College

Russia, x, 171, 187n5. *See also* Soviet Union

Rwanda, 187n5

safe sex, 27, 67–78, 111, 112, 119*t*, 123*t*, 124, 166

safety: of elderly people, 146–147; of RCSIP and RSIHM students, 22, 23, 28, 82, 106, 174–175; and social capital, 145

St. Basil's Free People's Clinic (Englewood neighborhood): community representatives at, 33, 41–43, 56, 63, 112; free services at, 31–32, 42, 60–61, 63; number of patient contacts at, 34; Peter DeGolia as volunteer at, 16, 18, 32–33; prenatal clinic at, 27, 34–36, 40–41, 43, 63, 119*t*, 121, 122*t*, 123, 167; RCSIP's work at, 30–43, 48, 50, 52, 53, 60–63, 76, 93, 102, 119*t*, 120*t*, 122*t*, 148, 165; Sue Thompson as volunteer at, 26, 27, 34–36, 40, 43

St. Bernard's Hospital (Englewood neighborhood), 30

St. Joseph's Hospital (Chicago), 52

St. Pius Catholic Church (Pilsen neighborhood), 125, 167

Salvation Army Temple (Chicago), 167

SCHIP, 154

Schlaffer, Carrie, 19

Schoenberger, James A., 21, 54

School of Public Health (Berkeley, California), 53, 54

schools: AIDS prevention programs at, 68–72, 76, 78, 112, 119*t*, 124, 166; asthma education in, 86; health-related events at, 166, 167; obesity-reduction education in, 155, 156, 166, 167; sex education in, 71, 75, 155. *See also* medical education; universities

Schroeder, Steven, 2

Schweitzer, Albert, x

Schweitzer Fellows, ix–x, 103

Schwer, William, 19–20

science vs. service, in medical education, viii–ix, 3–5, 12, 24, 26–27, 38–39, 41, 55, 61–62, 77–78, 113, 128*t*, 133, 135, 139, 149–151, 159, 161–162, 182

Secretary of Health and Human Services Award for Innovation in Health Promotion and Disease Prevention, 36, 43, 75

Sehagal, Niraj Laksham, 53–55

Sen, Amartya, 96

Serbia, 97, 106

service: "learning by doing" through
voluntary, xi, 8–10, 13, 15–17, 20, 28, 30,
36–41, 46–47, 50–55, 57–60, 62, 100,
108–111t, 112–117, 130, 133–134, 158;
Robert Coles on, 9, 12, 15; vs. science in
medical education, viii–ix, 3–5, 12, 24,
26–27, 38–39, 41, 55, 61–62, 77–78, 113,
128t, 133, 135, 139, 159, 161–162, 182;
staying power of the call of, 161–71. *See
also* community service; humanism; Rush
Community Service Initiatives Program
(RCSIP)
Service Employees International Union
(SEIU), 154
sex education, 71, 75, 78, 124, 155
sexually transmitted diseases, 19, 124, 134,
145, 167. *See also* AIDS/HIV
Shapiro brothers, 32
Shea, Patty, 21
Shipler, David, 144
Shiprock (New Mexico), 40
sickle-cell anemia, 122, 123t
Sinnott, Jessica, 169
skin infections, 121
Skinner, B. F., 6
"slow medicine," 20, 38
Small, Albion, 188n6
SMCHHR track (proposed, for medical
education), 183–186
smoking, 122, 123t, 124, 156, 185
social capital, 145, 170
Social Medicine, Community Health, and
Human Rights Curriculum (proposed),
181–186
The Social Order of the Slum (Suttles), 80
social responsibility: in Cuba, 103–104;
international, as physicians' role, 98, 163;
as key component of medical
professionalism, 140–153, 159–160,
170–171, 186; as physicians' role, 3, 28,
39–40, 50–51, 53–55, 58–59, 76–77, 105,
112–116, 123, 130–131, 135, 137,
143–153, 170–171; RCSIP's demonstration
of, for medical education, 137–152. *See
also* community service
social status (class), 37, 110, 113–114, 136,
137, 143, 185; health effects of, x, xi, 5, 8,
9, 17, 18, 20, 26, 34, 37–41, 45–47, 53–55,
57–58, 76, 83–85, 87, 92–95, 99, 110,

112–113, 122–123, 131, 134–136, 138,
143–146, 157, 171, 184; of medical
students, 13, 14, 23, 39, 82, 125, 169. *See
also* poverty
Society of Teachers of Family Medicine, 38
sociocultural determinants of health, x, xi,
5, 8, 9, 17, 18, 20, 26, 34, 37–41, 45–47,
53–55, 57–58, 76, 83–85, 87, 92–95, 99,
110, 112–113, 122–123, 131, 134–136,
138, 143–146, 157, 171, 184. *See also*
social responsibility
The Sociological Imagination (Mills),
6–7
sociology, 2, 3, 26, 80, 136, 149, 155, 157,
182, 185, 188n6; Eckenfels's study of, 6–8;
tools of, 28
sonograms, 35
Sontag, Susan, 78
Sophie Davis State University (New York),
182
South Africa, 102–103, 106, 163
Soviet Union, 7. *See also* Russia
Soweto (South Africa), 102
Spanish language, 20, 44–46, 53, 63–64,
122, 125
The Spirit Catches You and You Fall Down
(Fadiman), 141
Stanford University, 75
Starr, Paul, 133
State Children's Health Insurance Plan
(SCHIP), 154
The Strategy of Preventive Medicine (Rose),
118
stress reduction, 122, 145–146
Stroger Hospital (formerly Cook County
Hospital), 25, 48, 49, 61, 63, 83, 85, 119t,
165, 167
strokes, 31, 145
"structural violence," x, xi
"Structure and Ideology in Medical
Education" (Bloom), viii, 4
students (at Rush Medical College):
academic performance of, 126–130, 128t,
186; attitudes of, toward involvement
in ambulatory care, 111–112;
backgrounds of, 13, 14, 23, 39, 82, 125,
169; and community asthma workers,
82–90, 111; in community-based health
clinics, 11, 15, 16, 18–20, 23, 24–27,

Edward J. Eckenfels is an emeritus professor in the Department of Preventive Medicine at Rush University Medical Center in Chicago. During more than thirty years at Rush, he has taught; conducted research; and developed programs in social medicine, community health, and medical education. He has been active in promoting voluntary community service and international health initiatives and as an advocate for the poor and disadvantaged.